F Cancer! Coloring Book!

With some inspiration too!

F is for Cancer, and it stands for FIGHT! FIGHT for your life! FIGHT for your health! May your battle be short, and your body be healthy!

Sending many positive vibes your way!

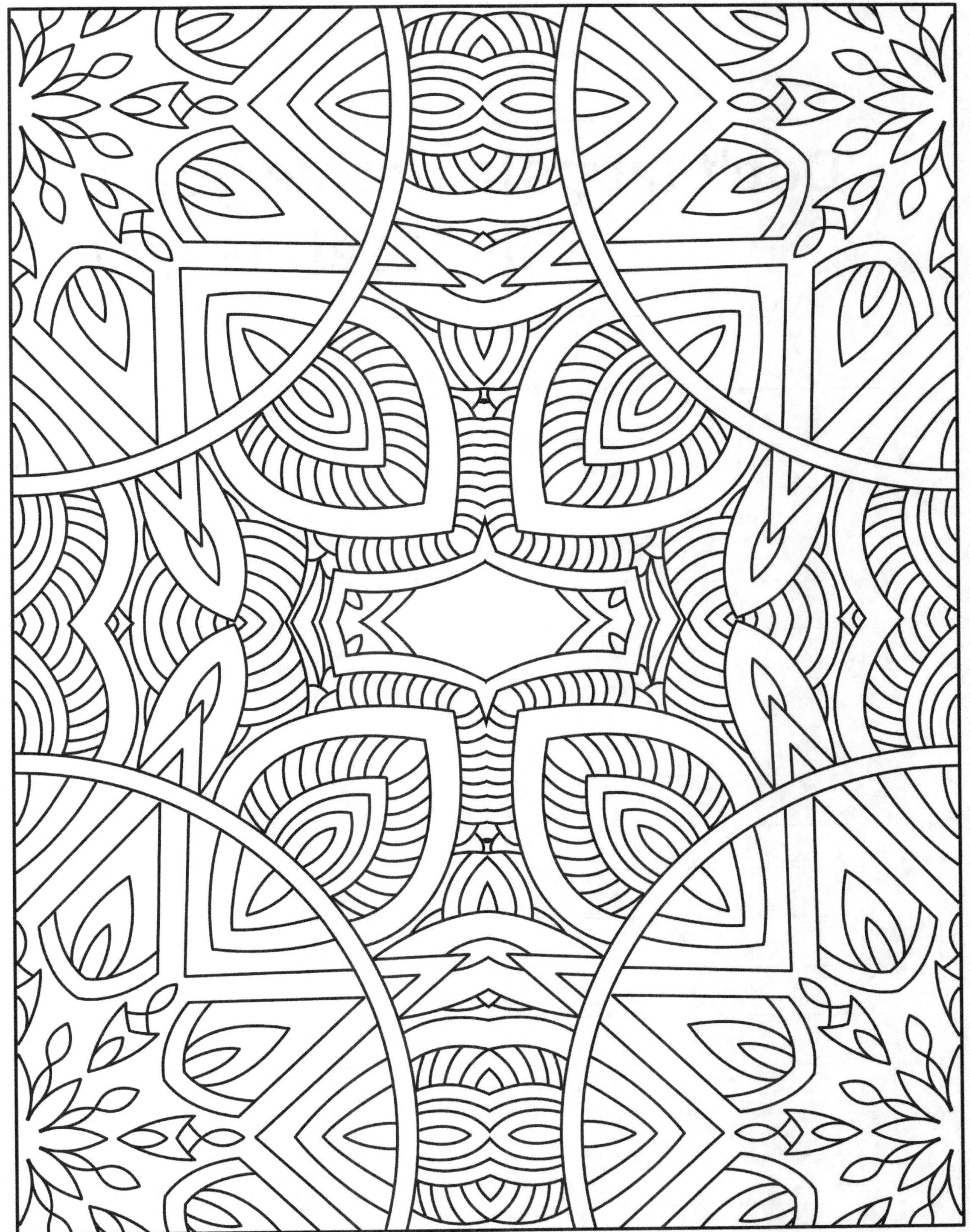

Don't let pain define you, let it refine you.

Tim Fargo

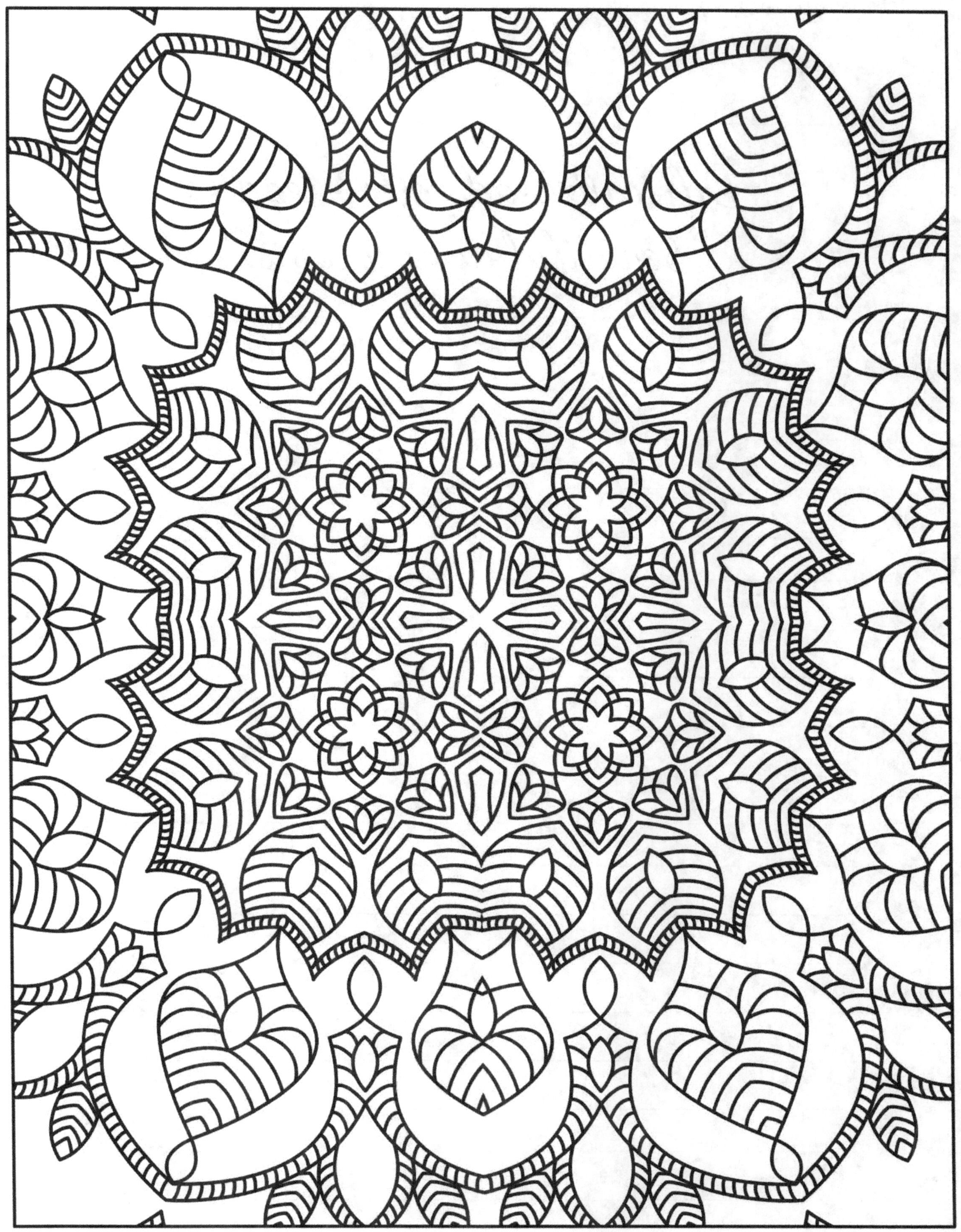

Difficult roads often lead to beautiful destinations.

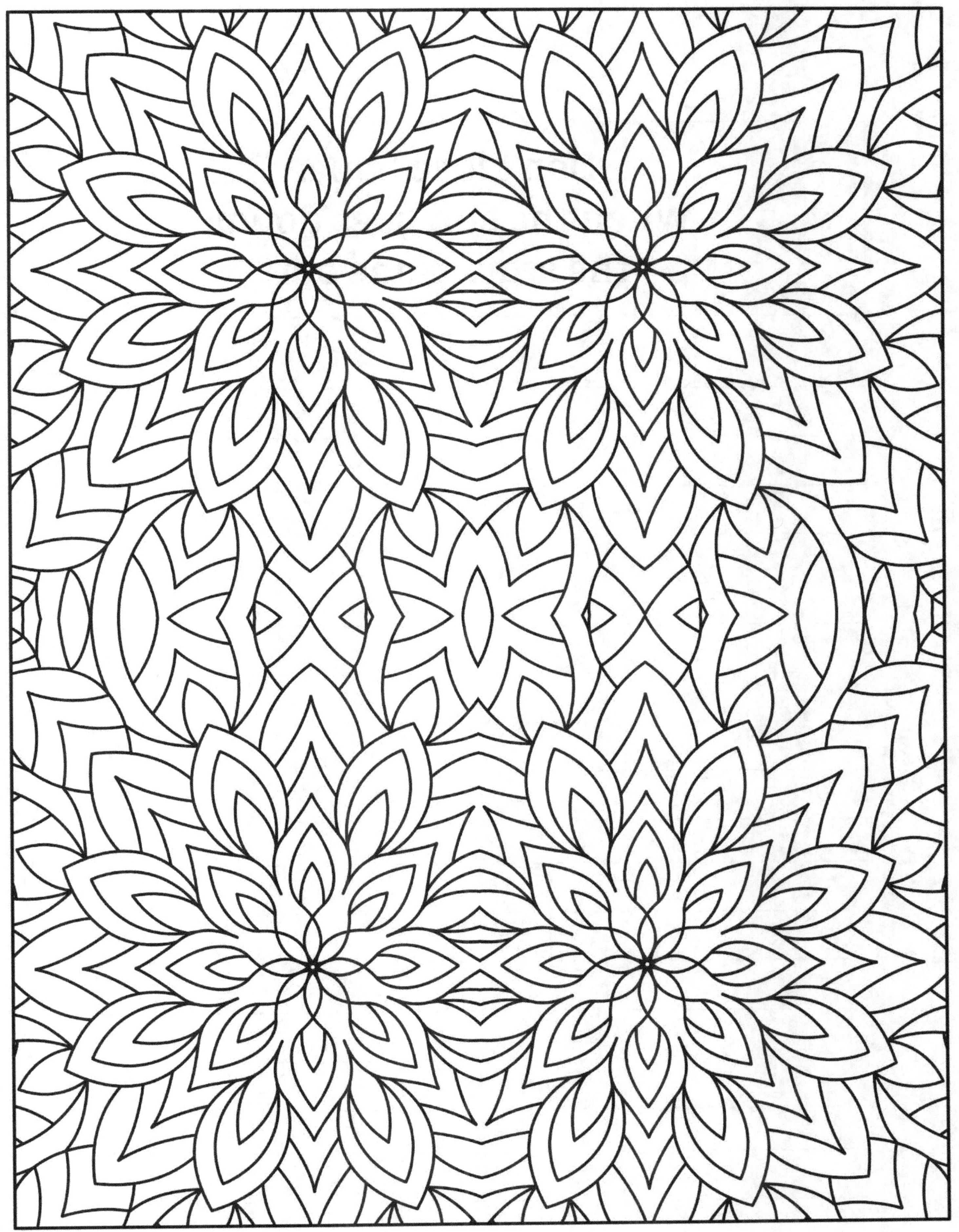

Don't lose hope.
When the sun goes down,
the stars come out.

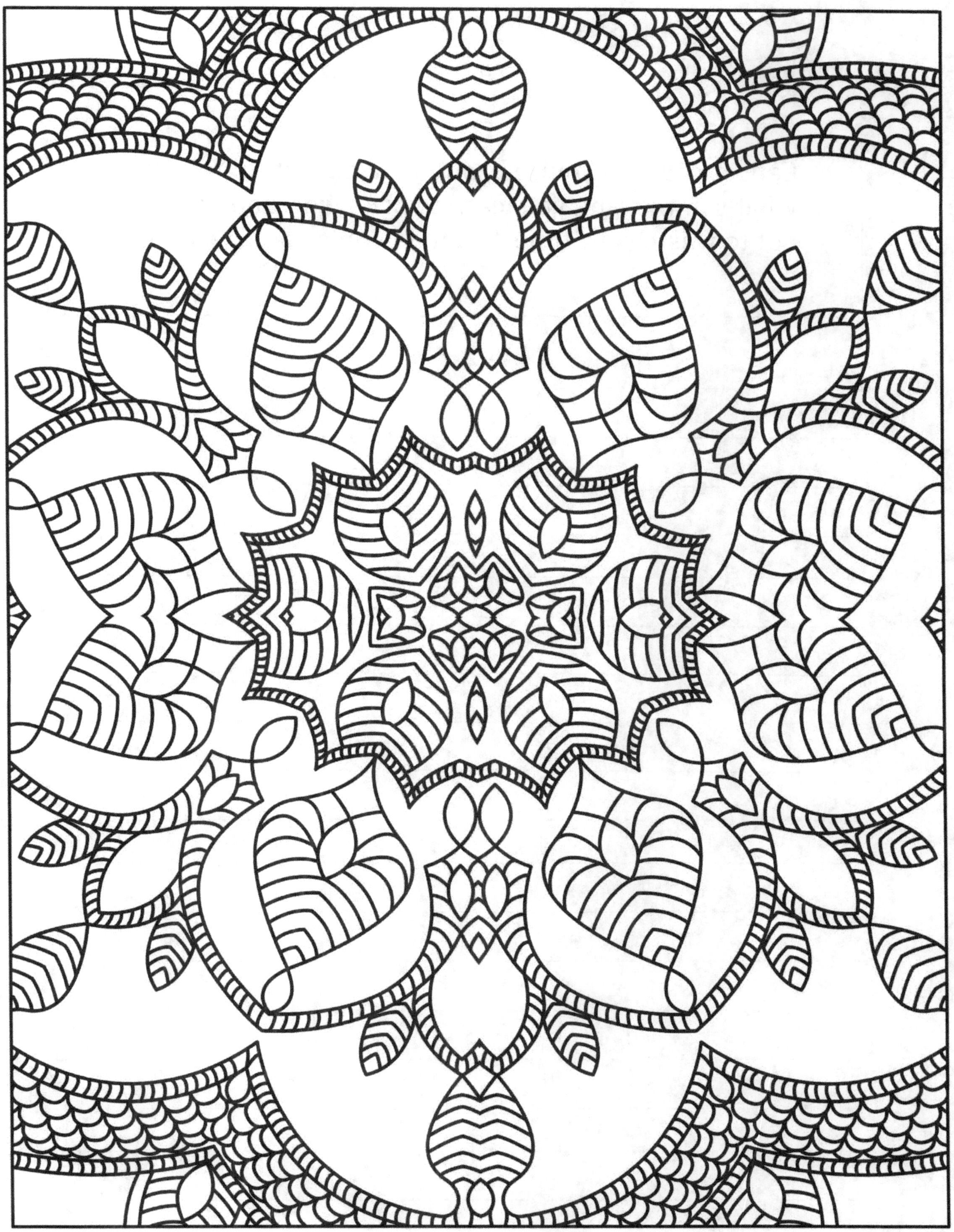

Cancer changes your life, often for the better. You learn what's important, you learn to prioritize, and you learn not to waste your time. You tell people you love them.

Joel Siegel

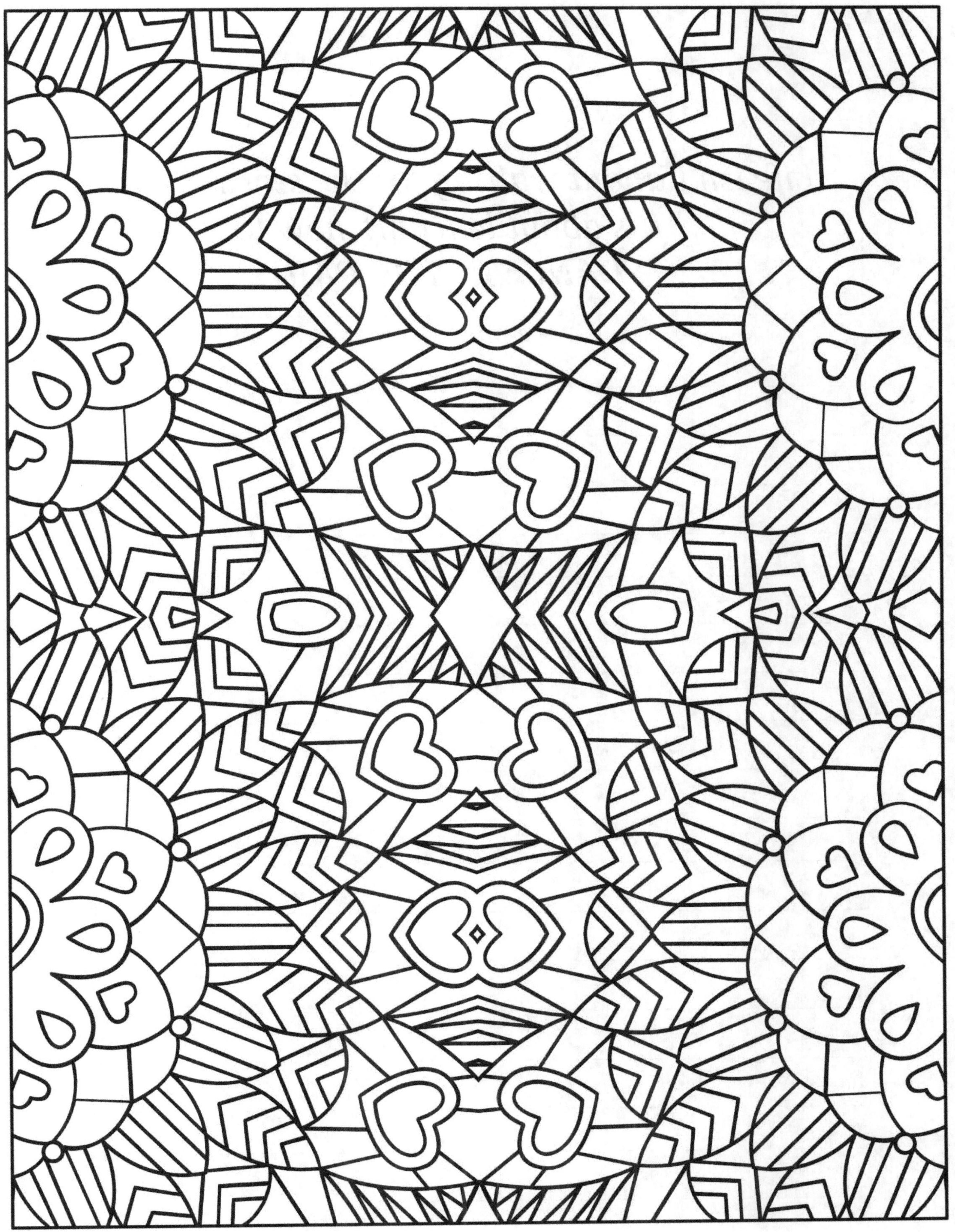

Life isn't about waiting for the storm to pass
It's about learning how to
DANCE IN THE RAIN

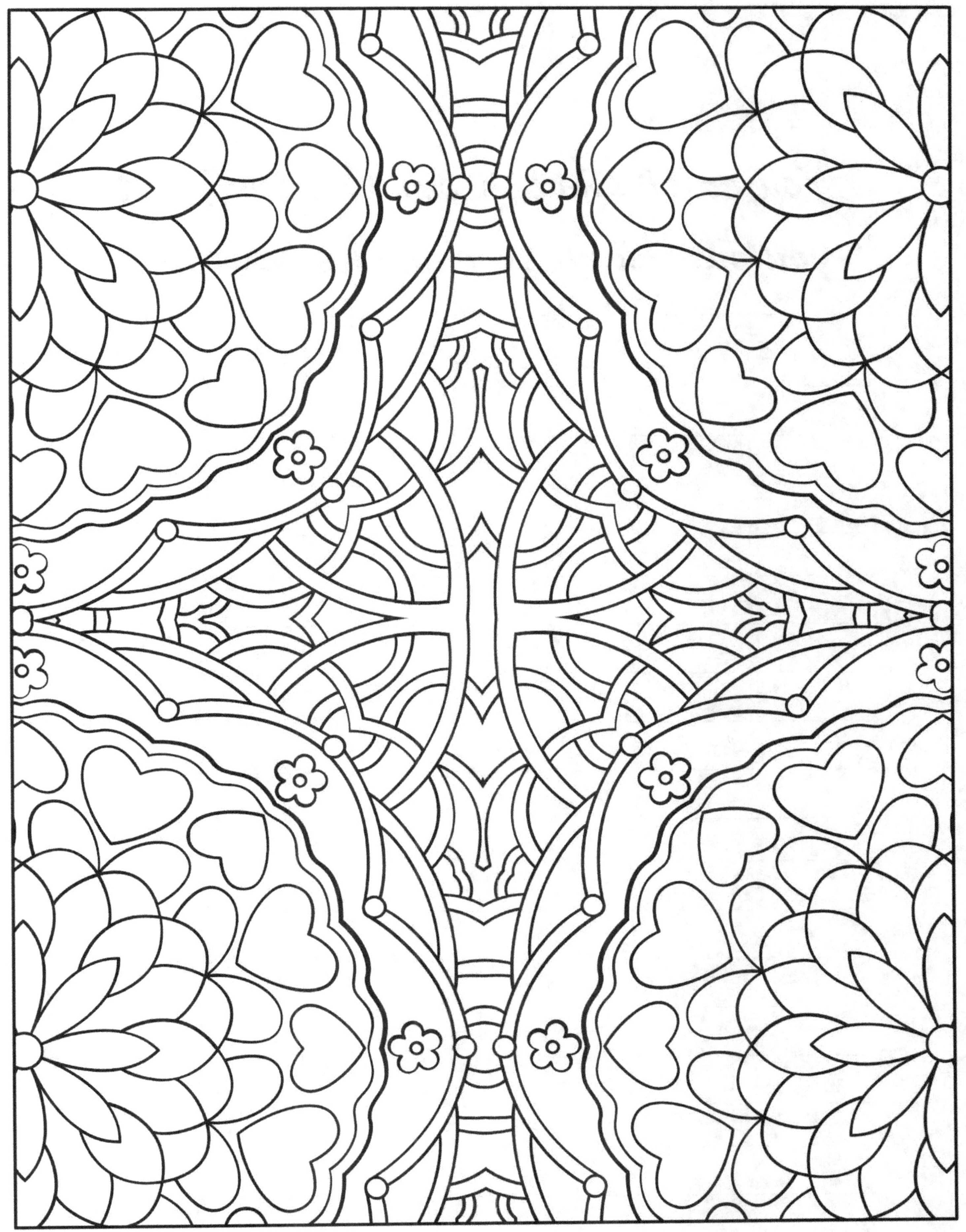

You can't smooth out the surf, but
you can learn to ride the waves.

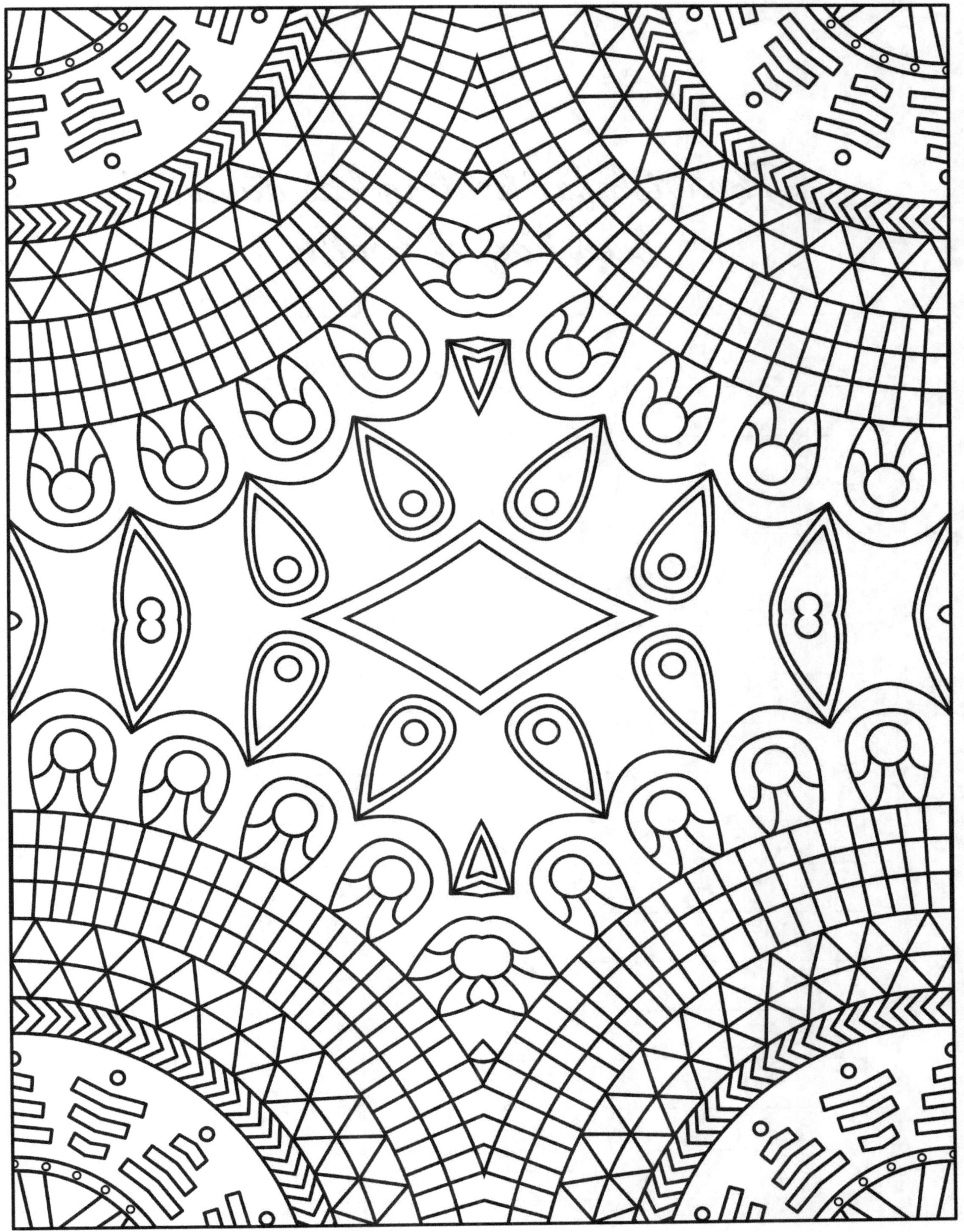

The wish for healing has always
been half of health.

Lucius Annaeus Seneca

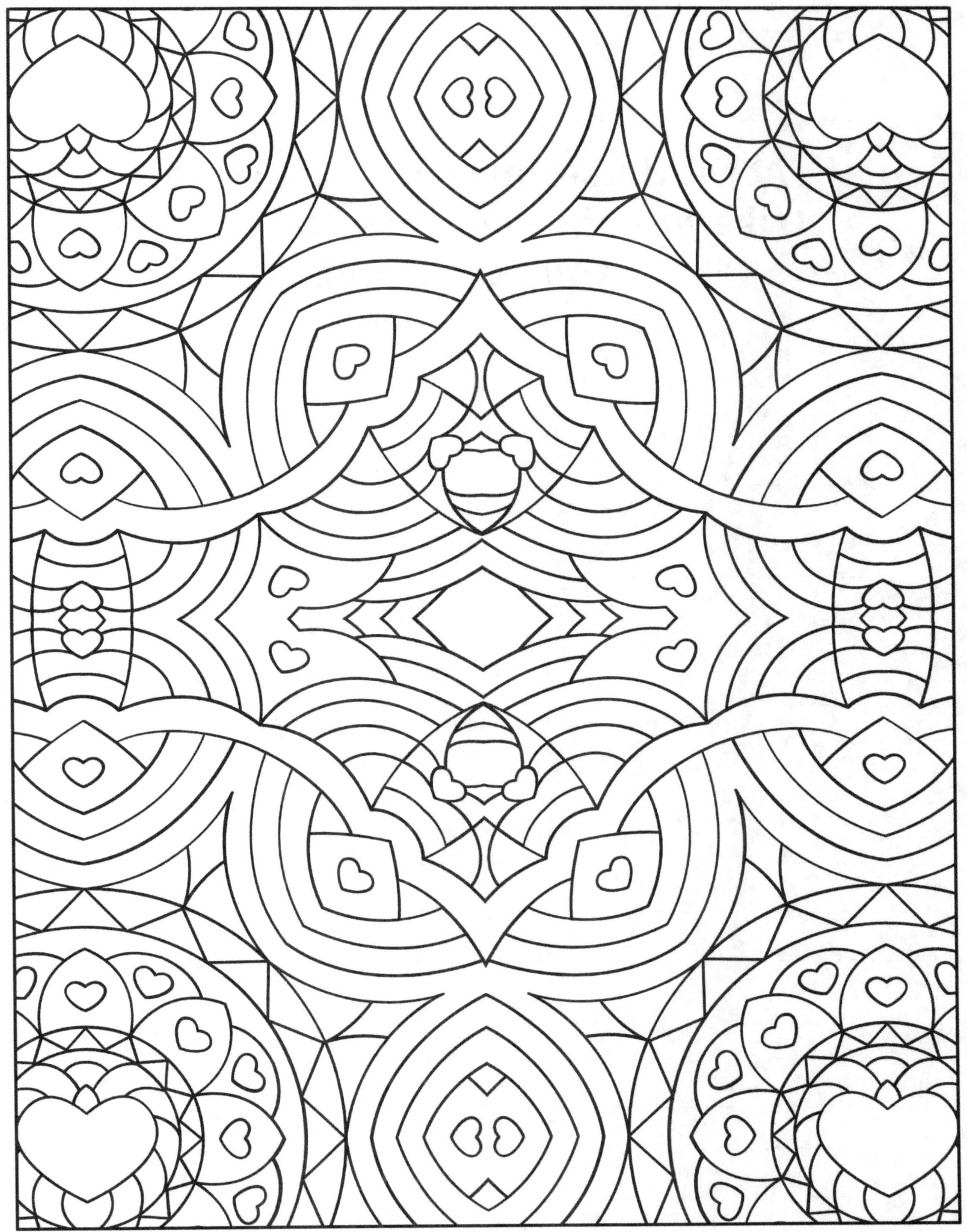

At the timberline where the storms strike with the most fury, the sturdiest trees are found.

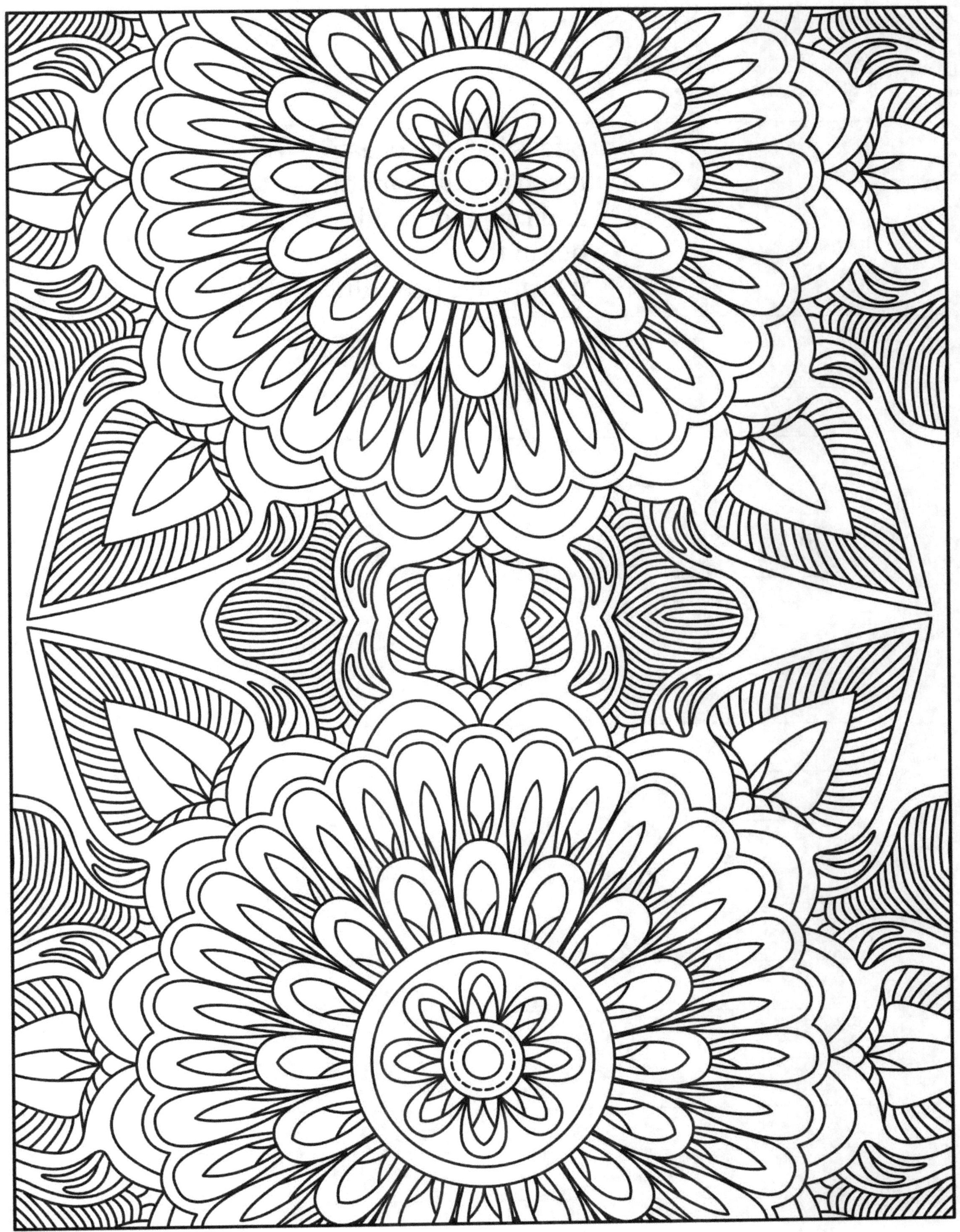

Life is like the ocean.
It can be calm or still,
and rough or rigid,
but in the end,
it is always beautiful.

Faith is daring to go beyond what
the eyes can see.

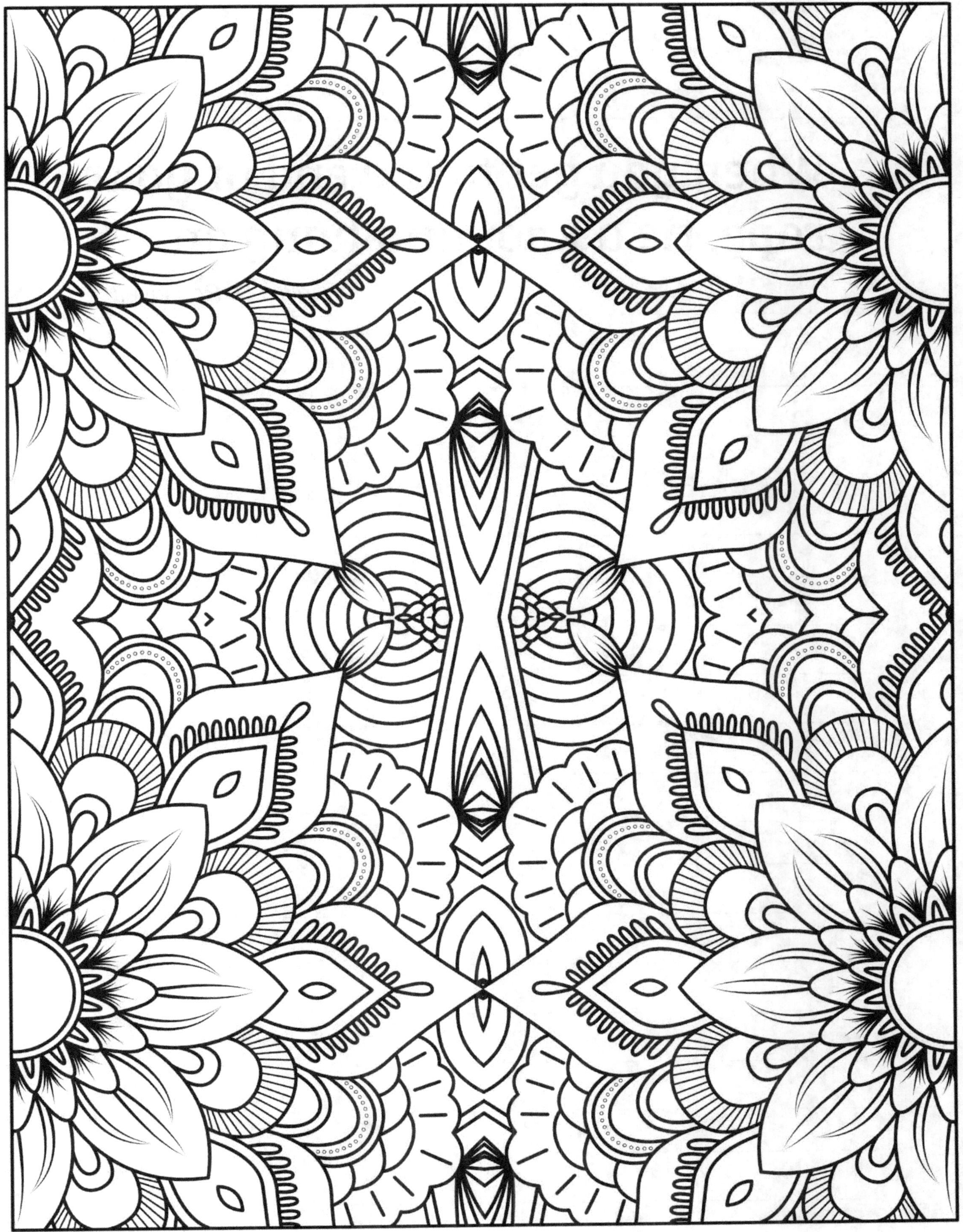

> # When you get to the end of your rope, tie a knot and hang on.
>
> *Franklin D. Roosevelt*

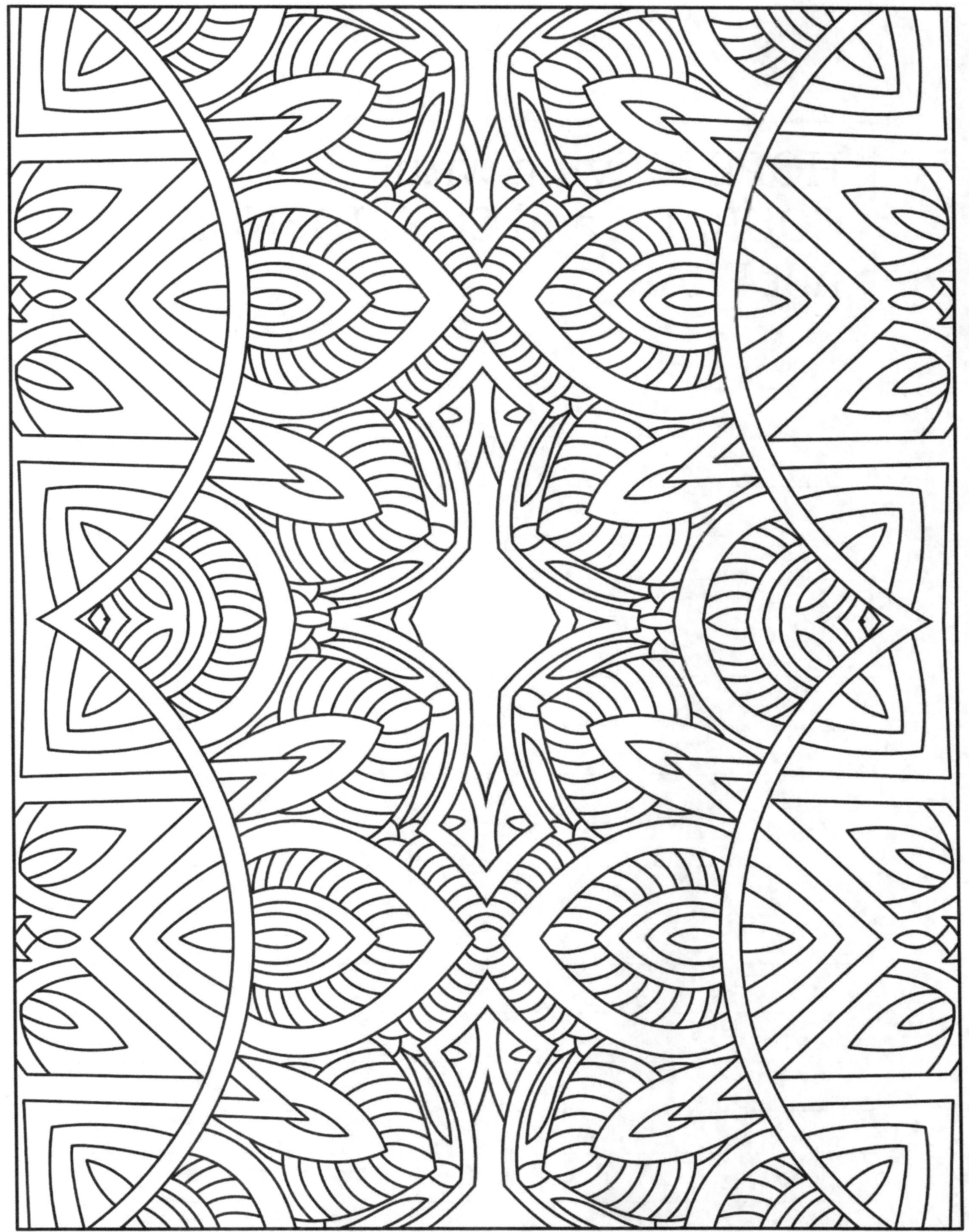

HOPE is living with
COURAGE and CONFIDENCE,
not FEAR.

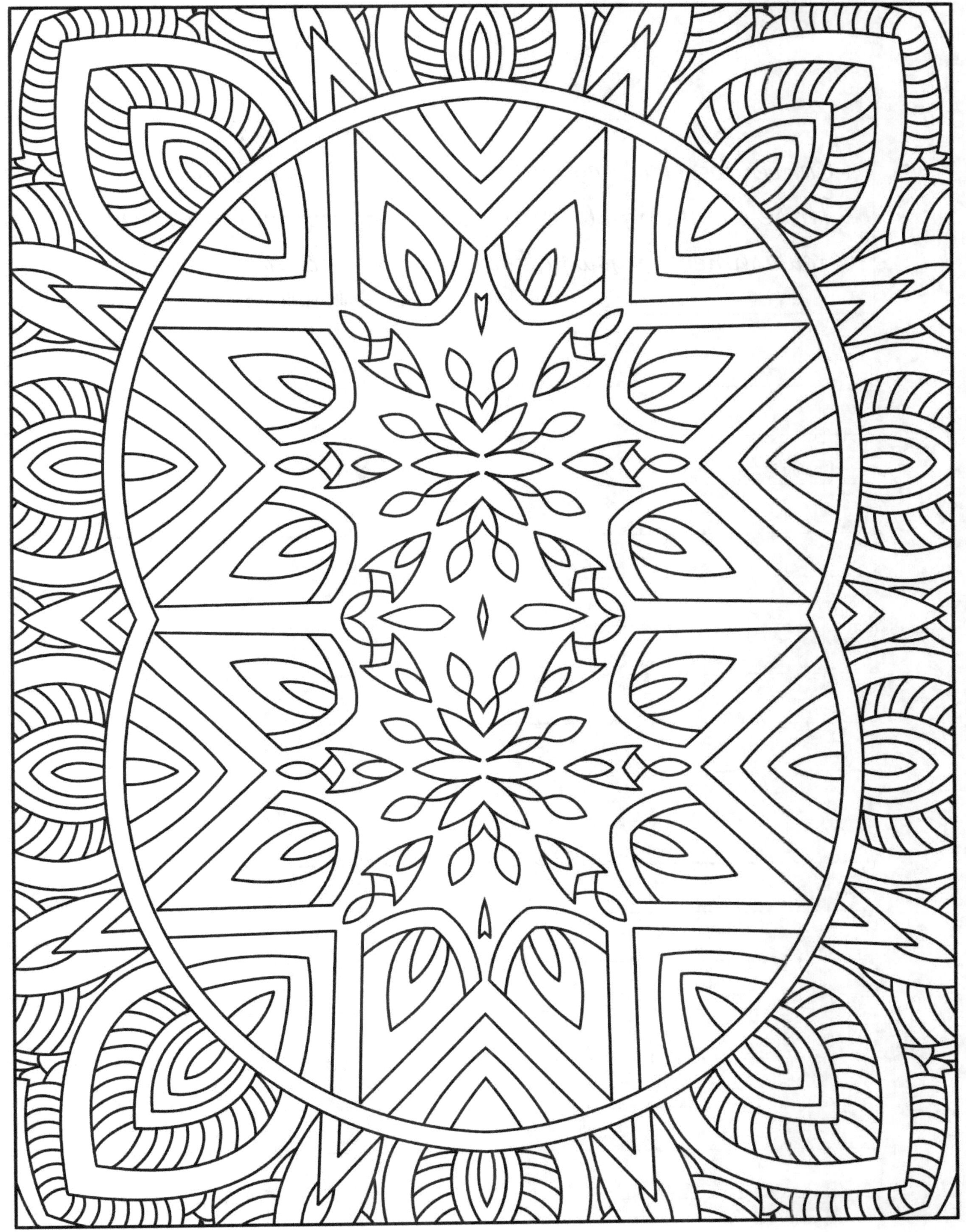

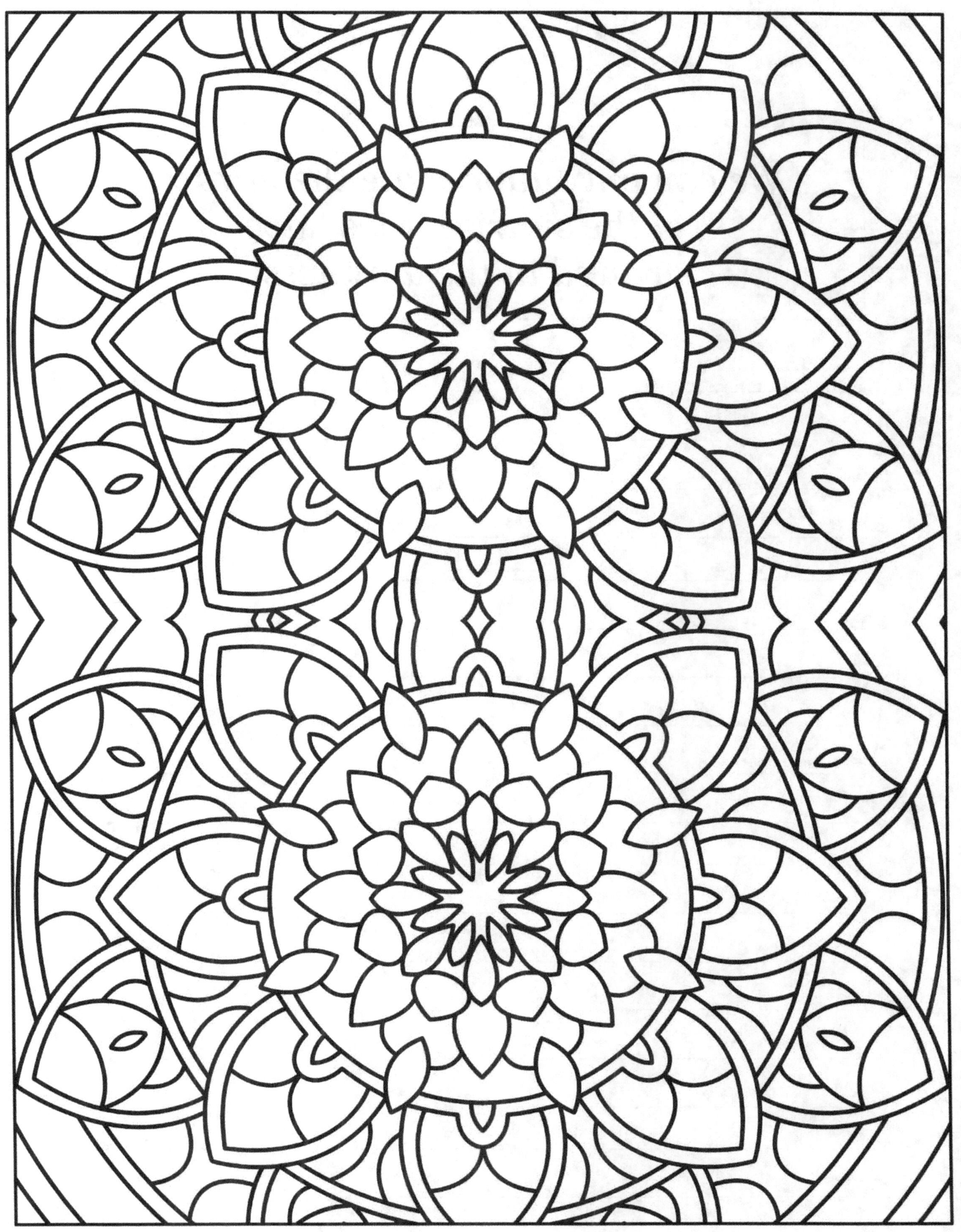

We can only appreciate the miracle
of the sunrise if we have
waited in the darkness.

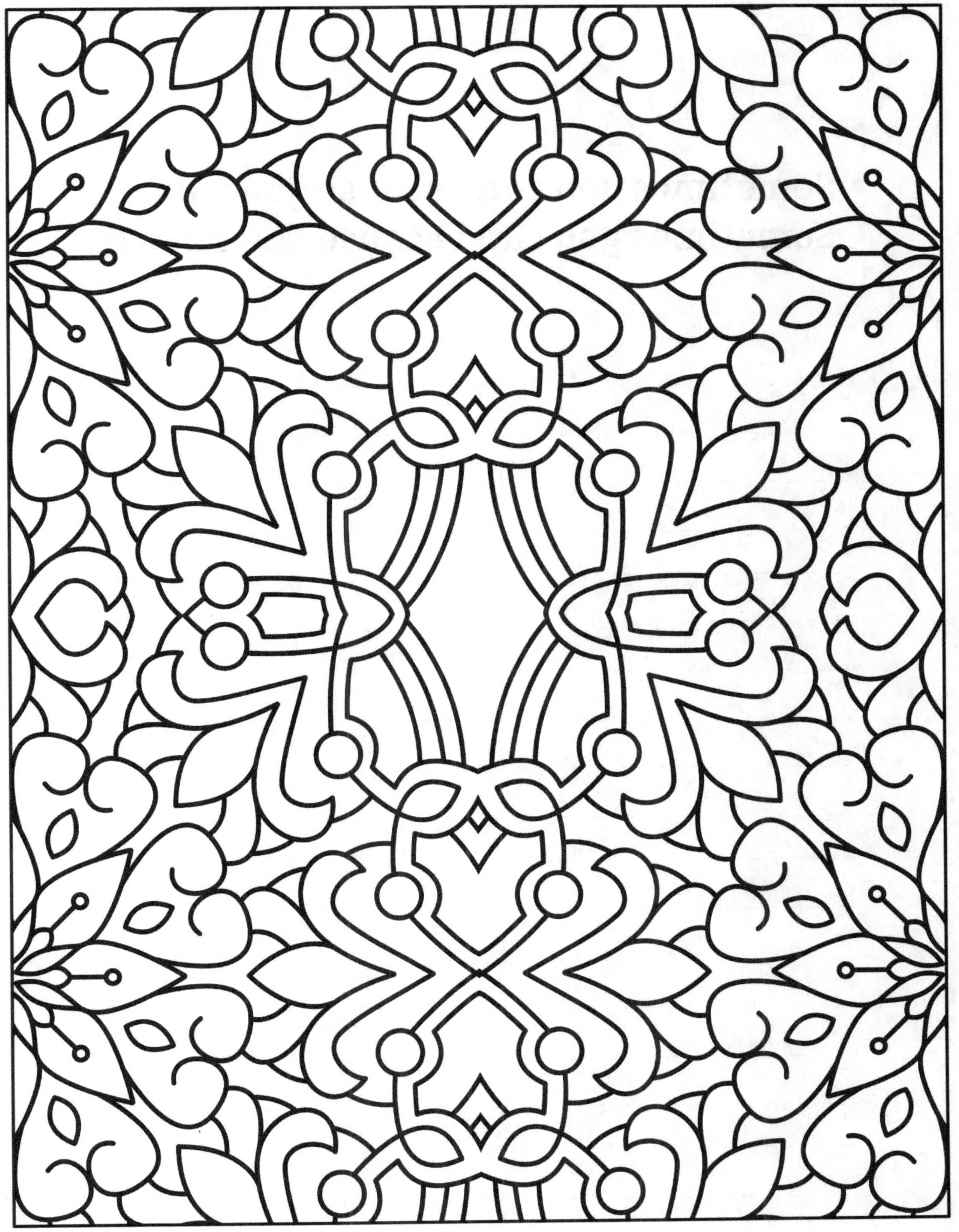

**Sometimes you can because you can.
Sometimes you can because you have to.**

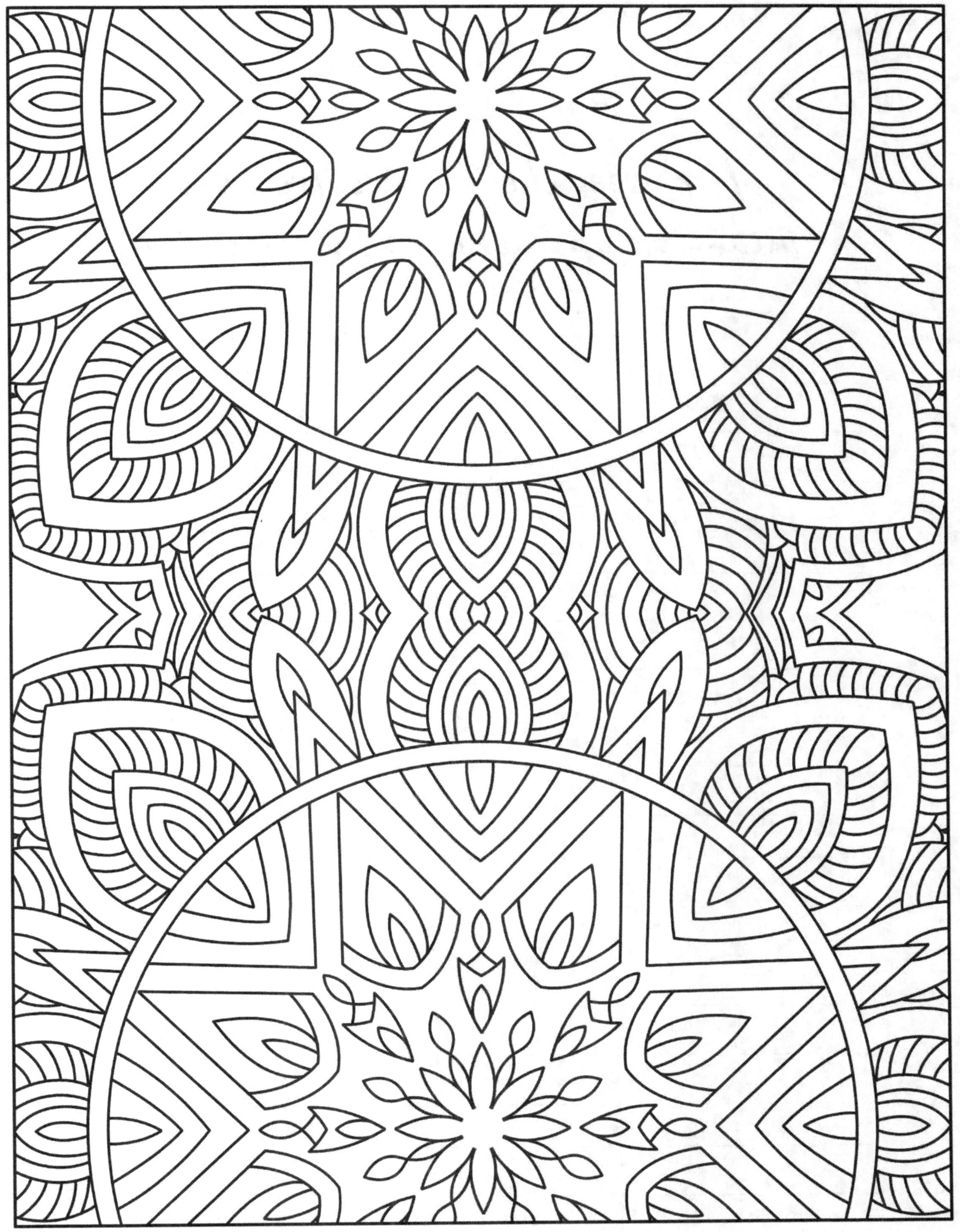

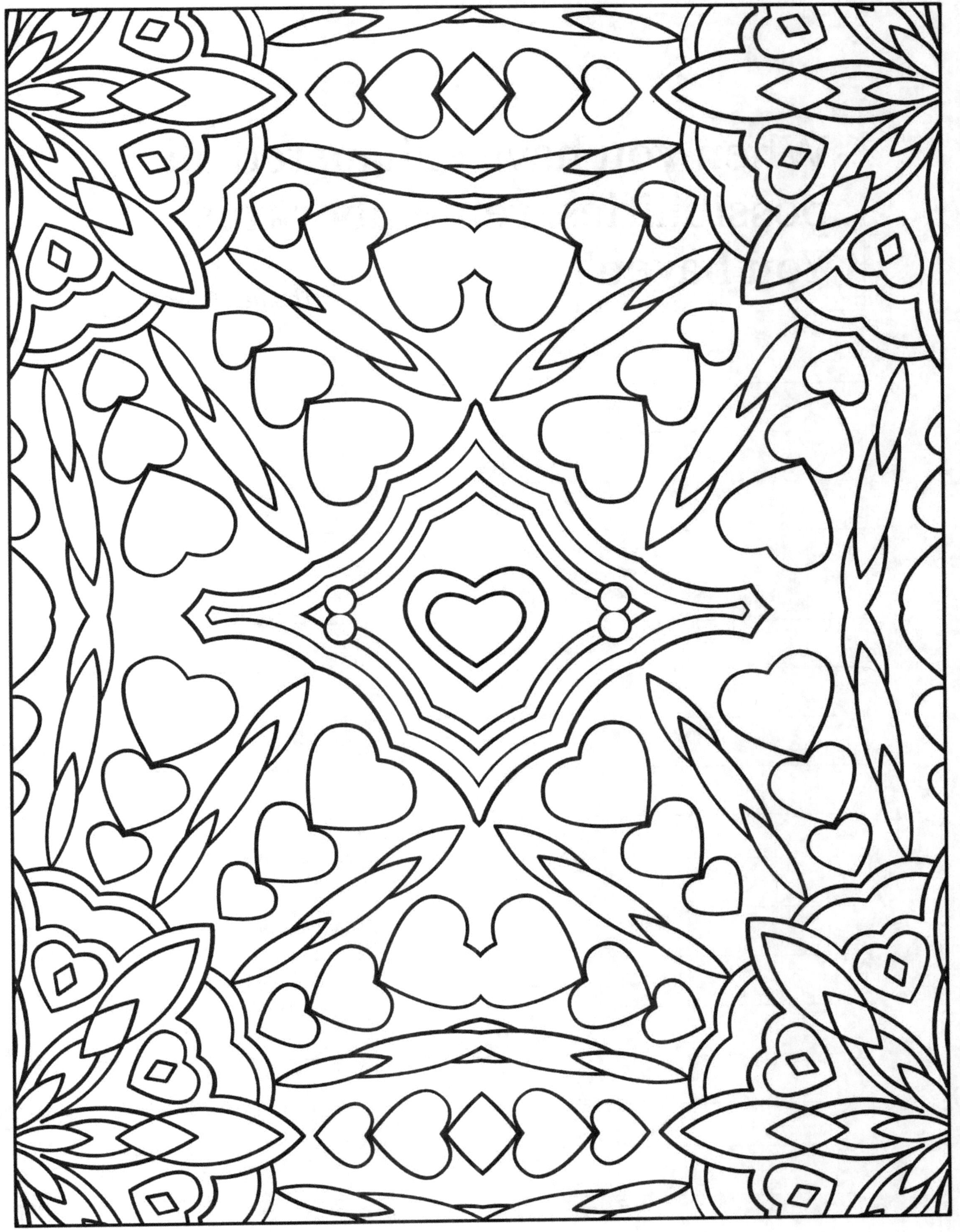

When you have exhausted all possibilities, remember this: You haven't.

Thomas Edison

Small Steps.... ***Everyday!***

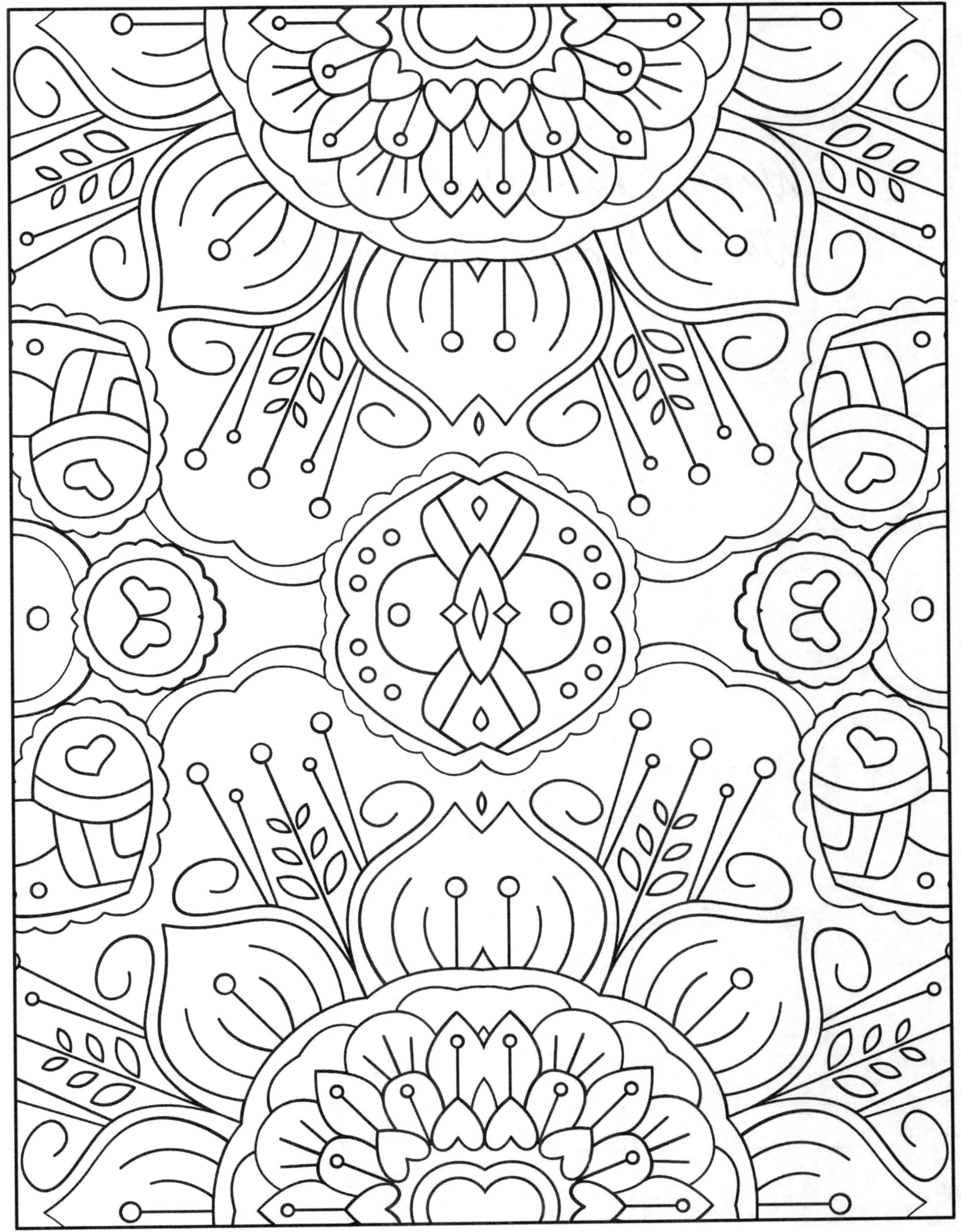

When it rains, look for rainbows
When it's dark, look for stars.

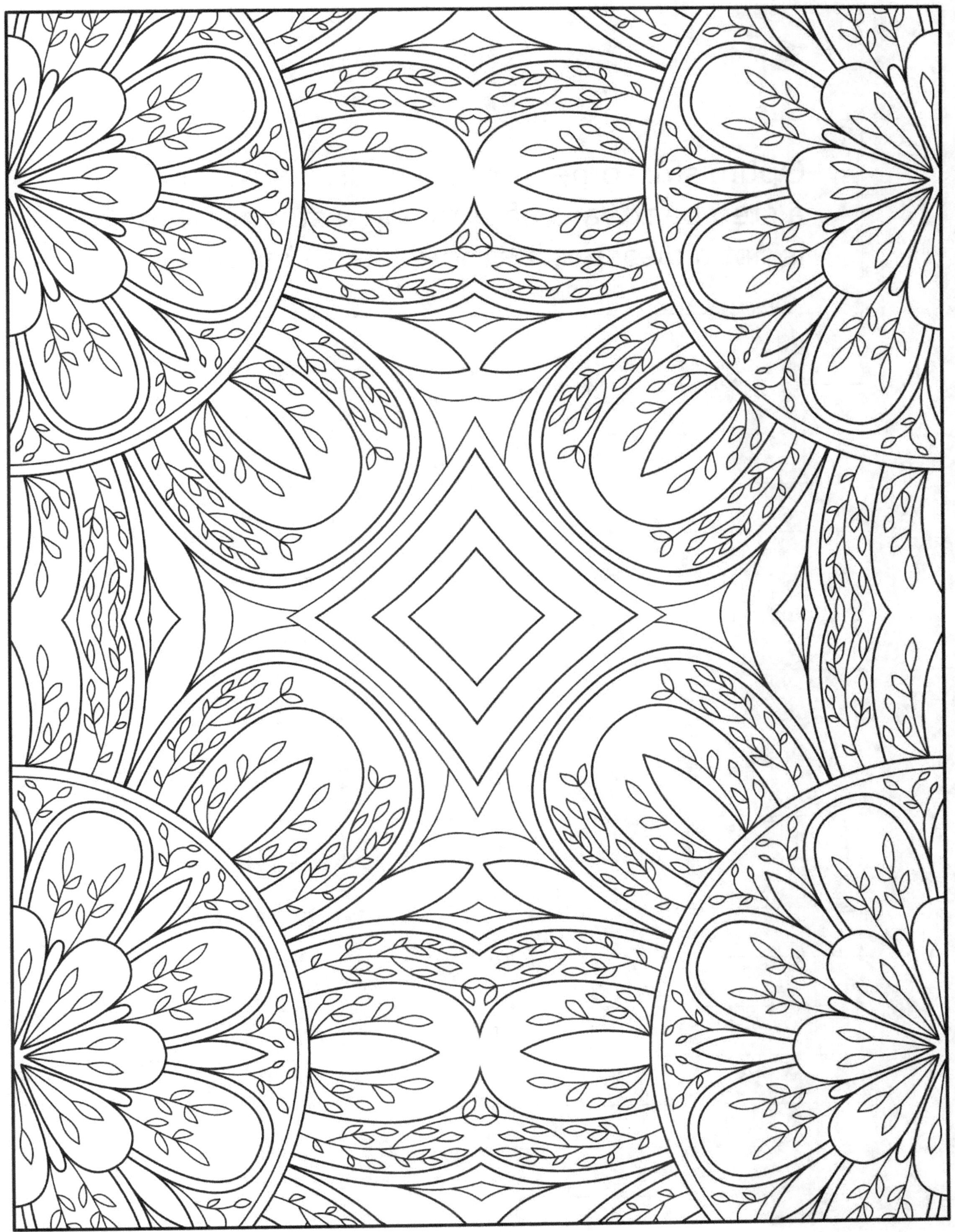

Optimism: someone who figures that taking a step backward after taking a step forward is not a disaster; it's more like a cha-cha.

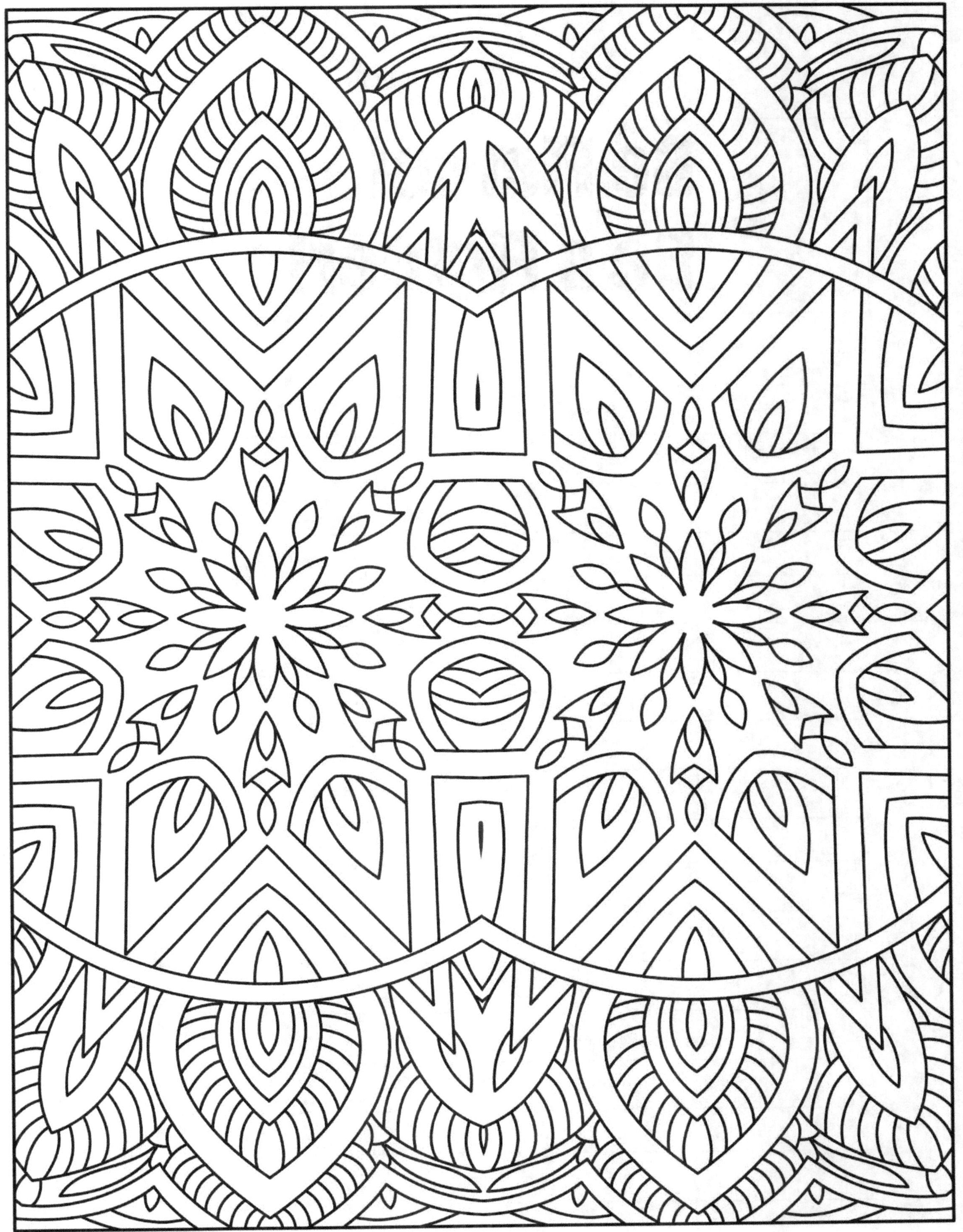

Be Fierce!
Be a Fighter!

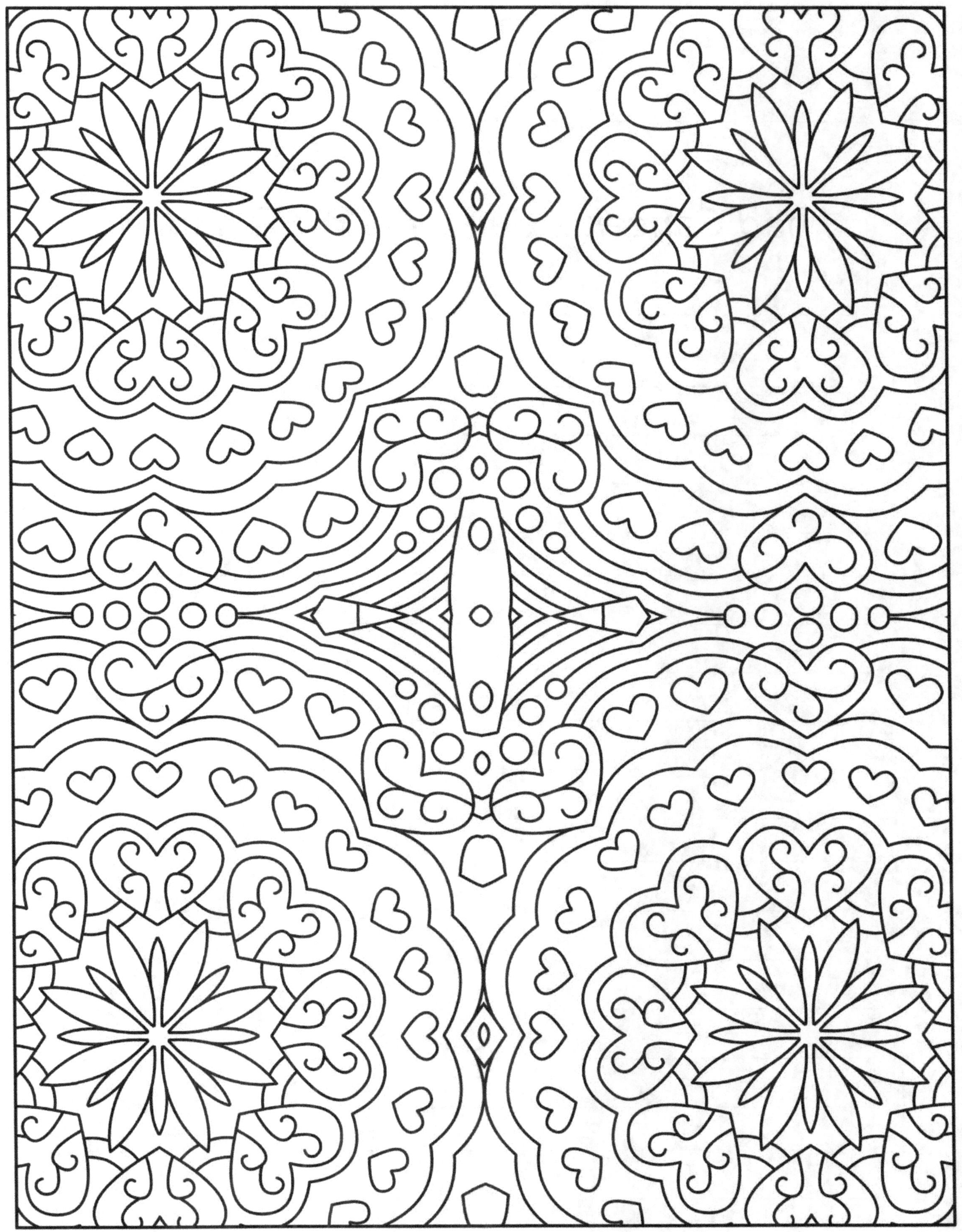

I had Cancer.... Cancer NEVER had ME!

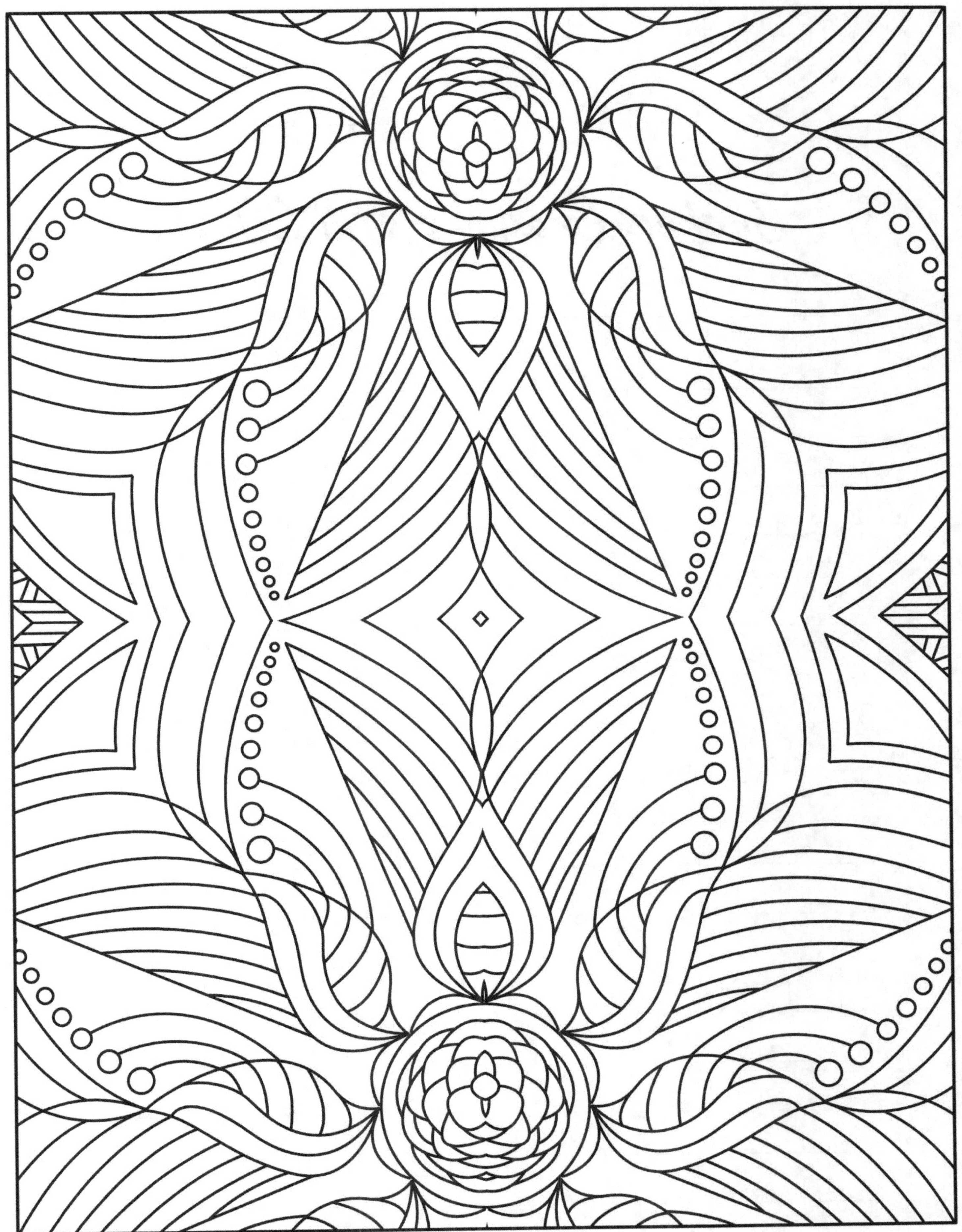

Broken Crayons still COLOR!

Cancer.... Is a Word!
Not a SENTENCE!

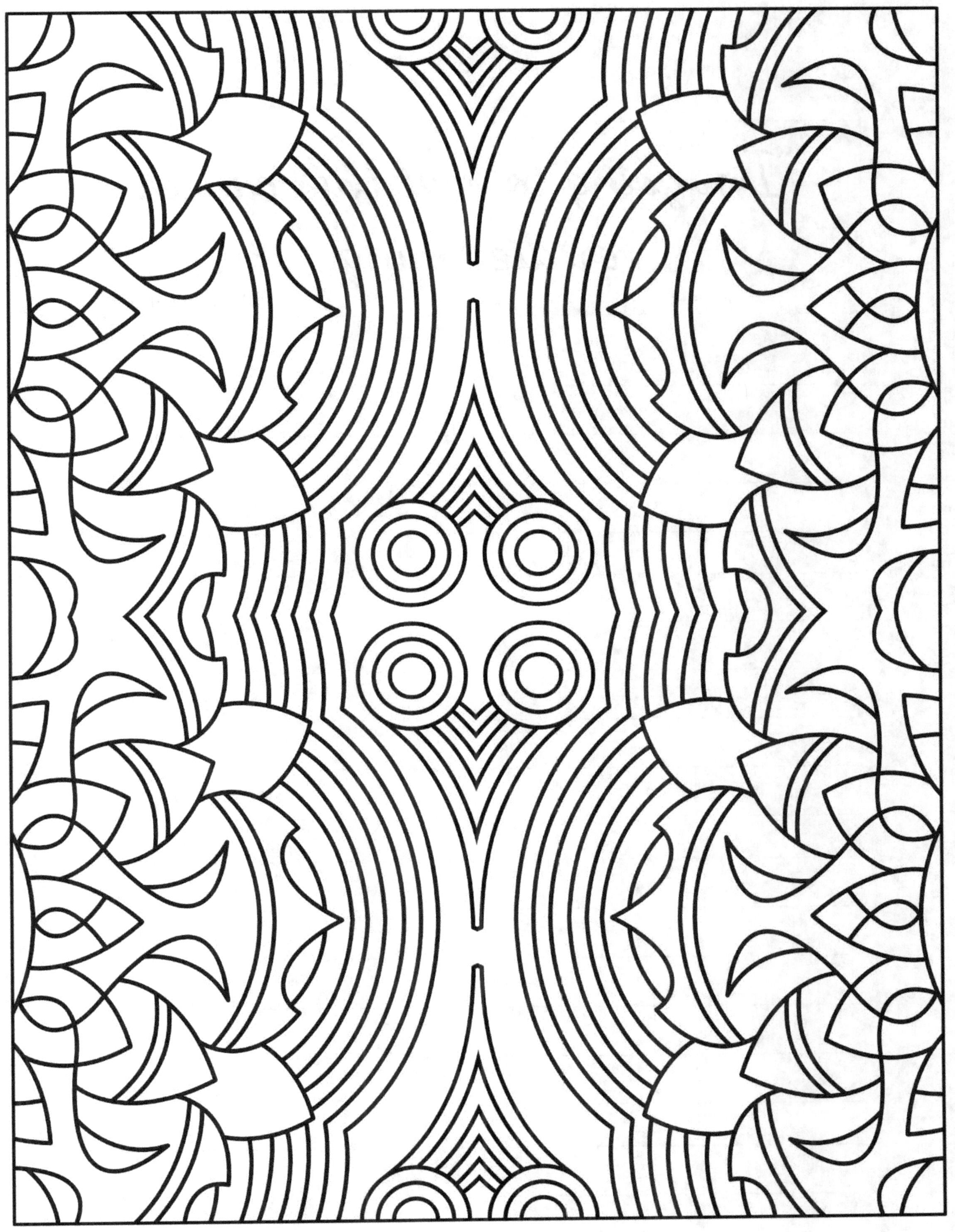

"I'm going to beat this cancer, or die trying."

Michael Landon

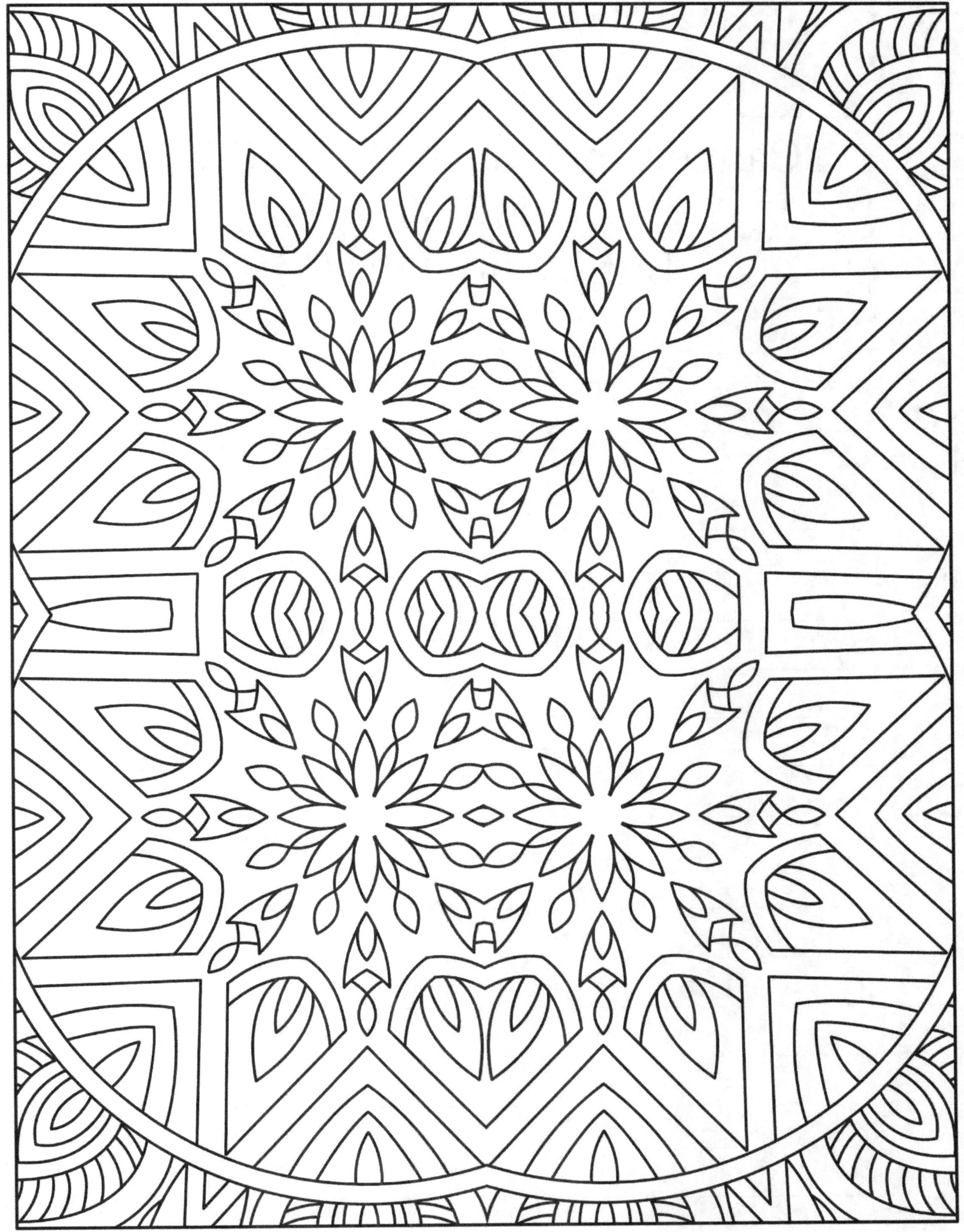

Cancer, may have STARTED the FIGHT,
but I will FINISH it!

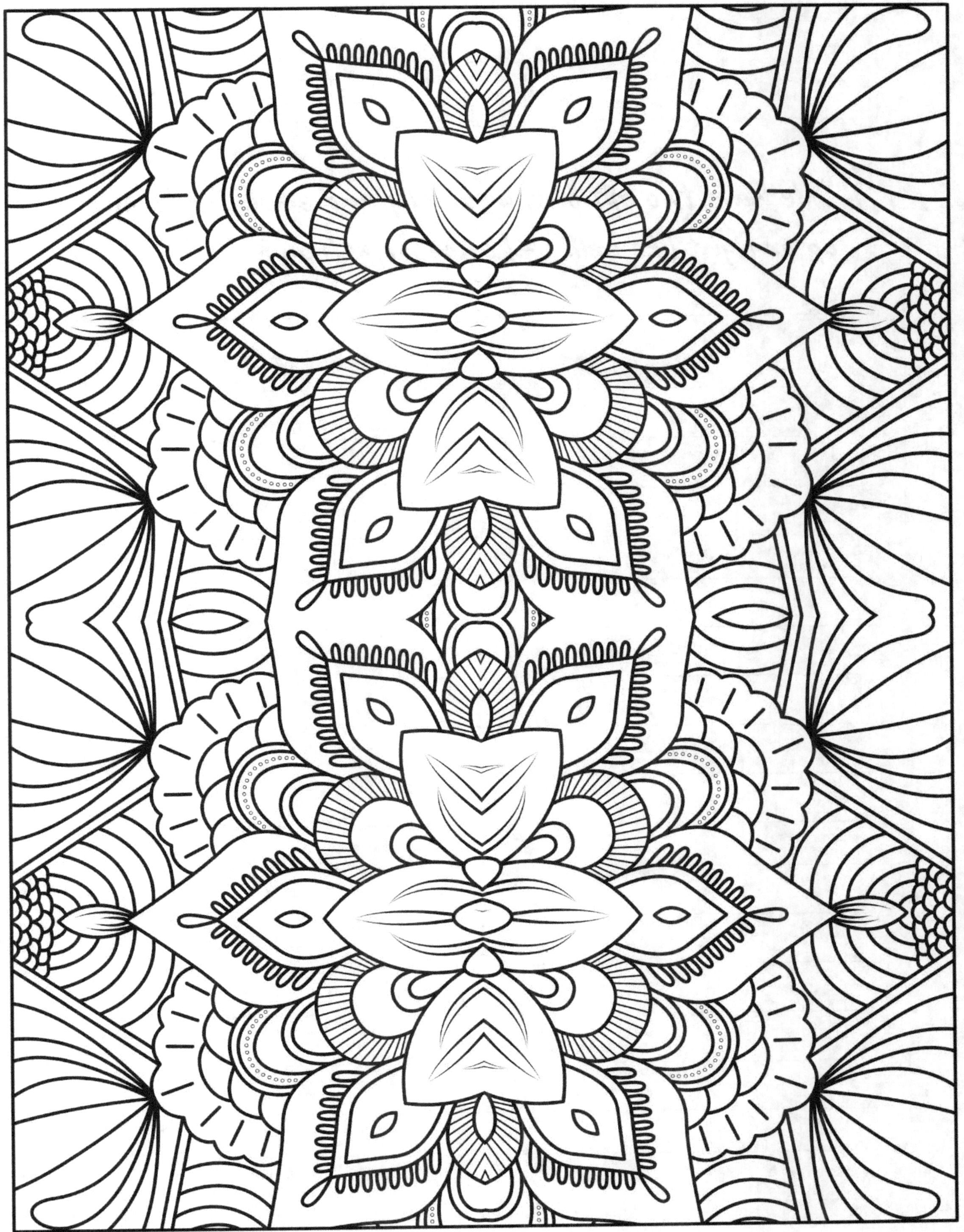

"We have two options, medically and emotionally: give up or fight like hell." – Lance Armstrong

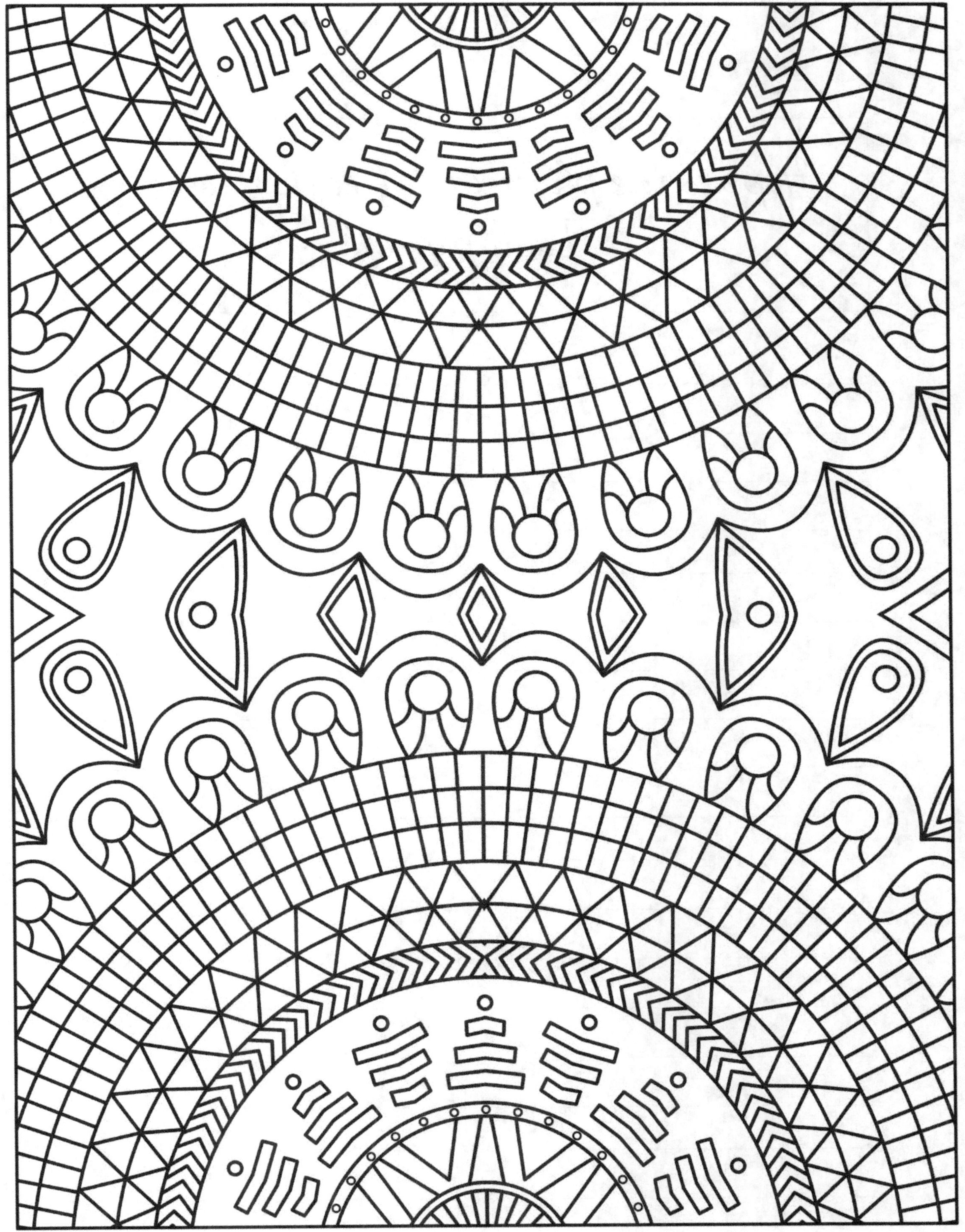

"Hope is the physician of each misery." —
Irish proverb

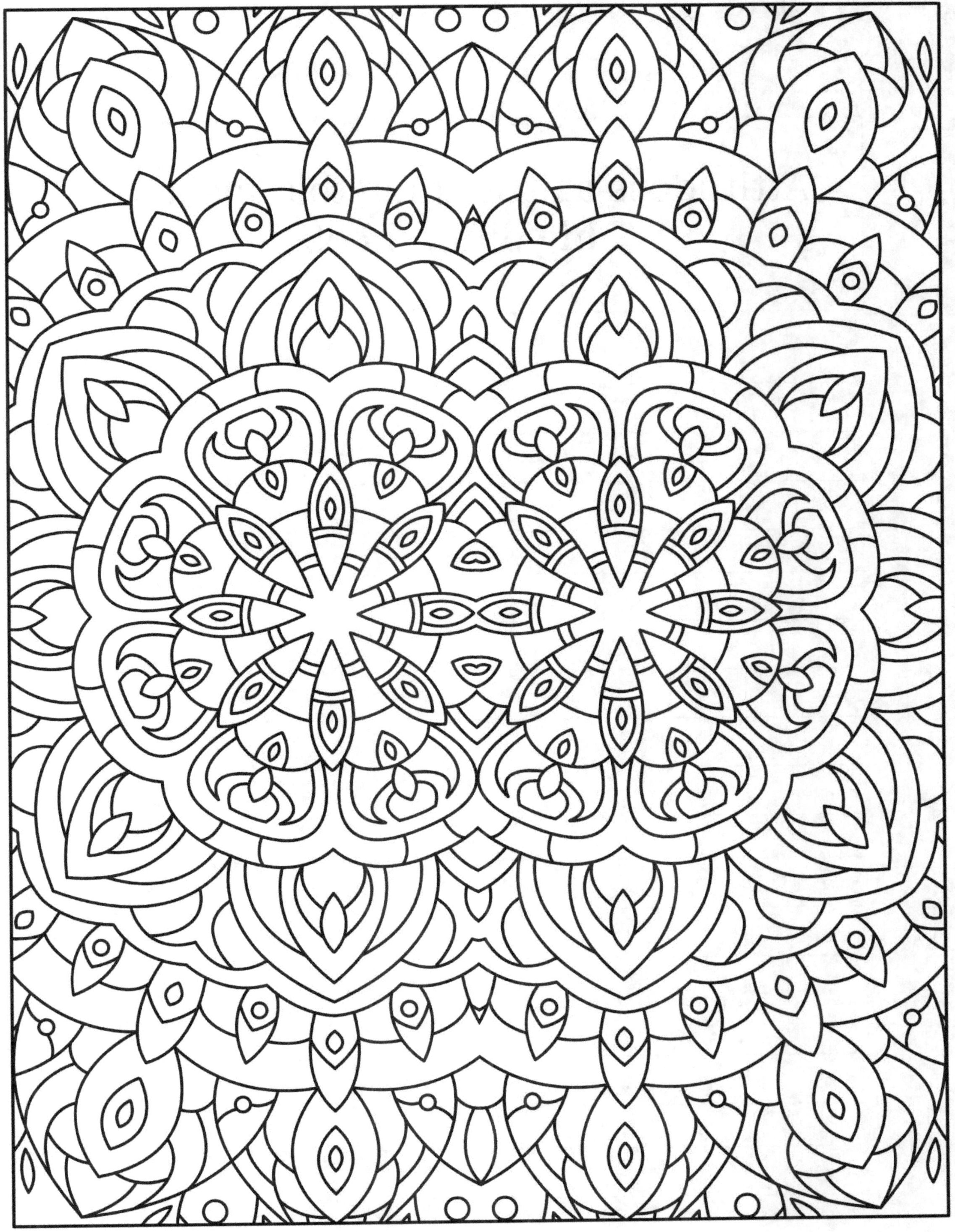

Attitude is a little thing that makes a **big** difference!

You never know how strong you are until being strong is the only choice you have.

Cayla Mills

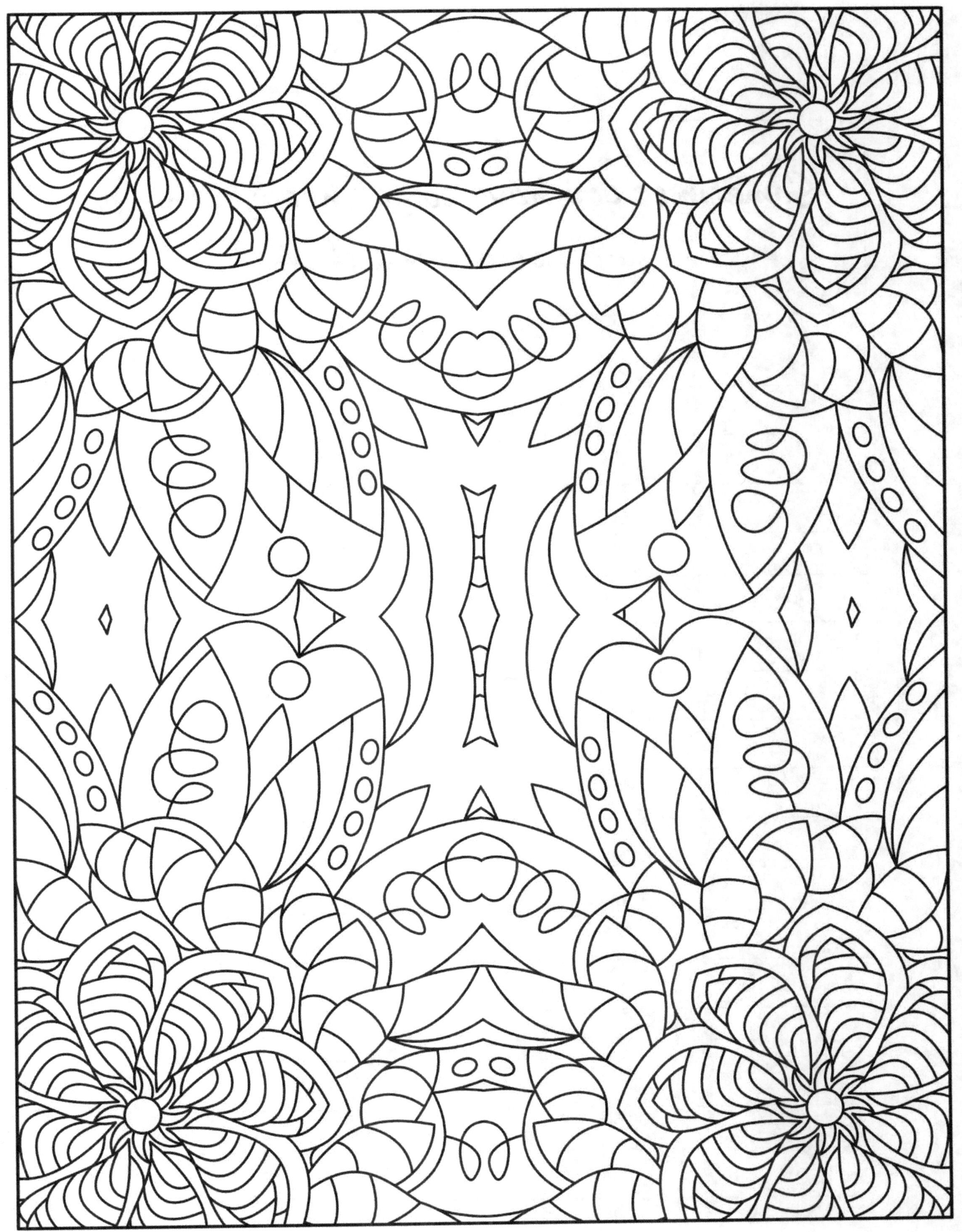

Sometimes you have to go through things and not around them.

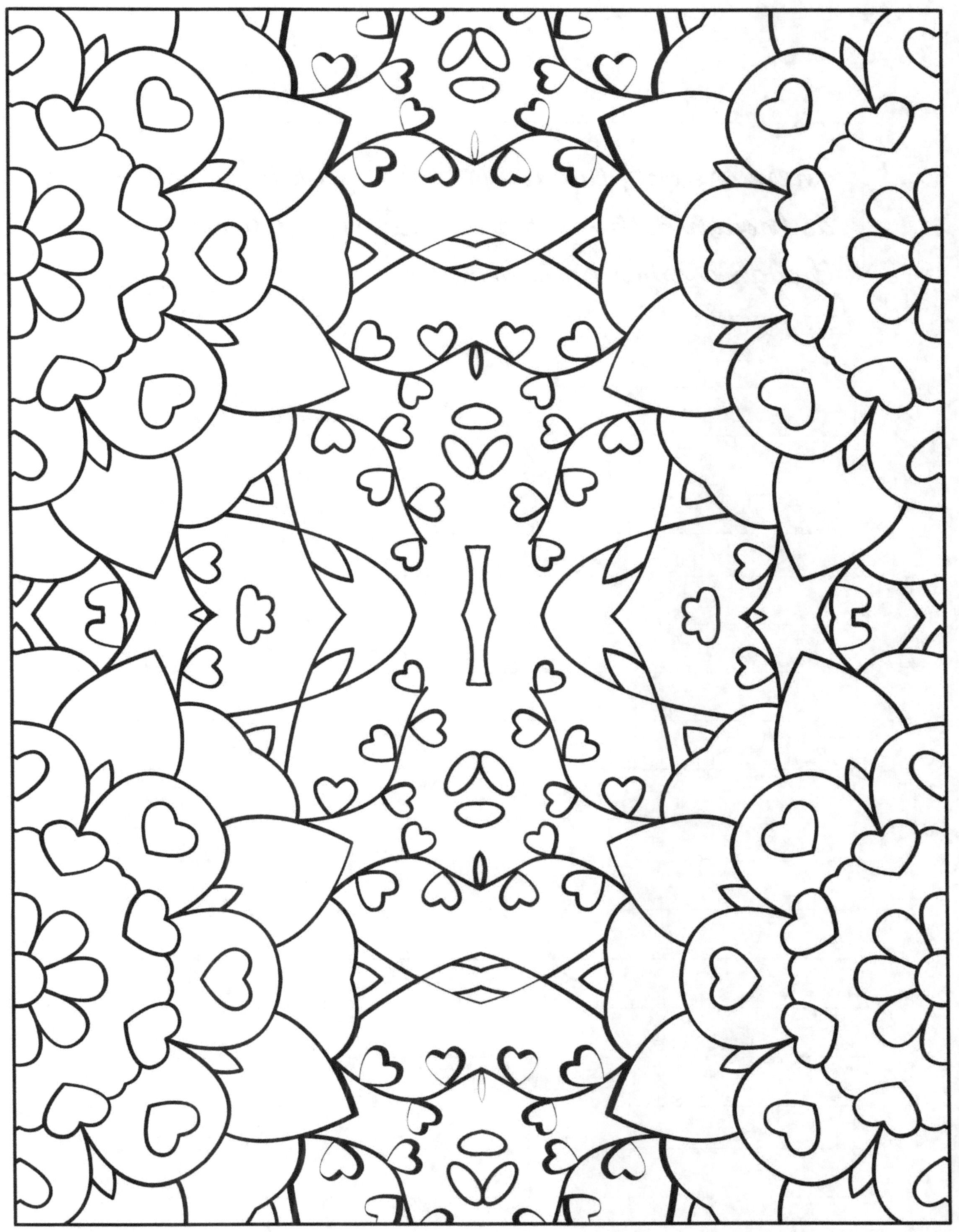

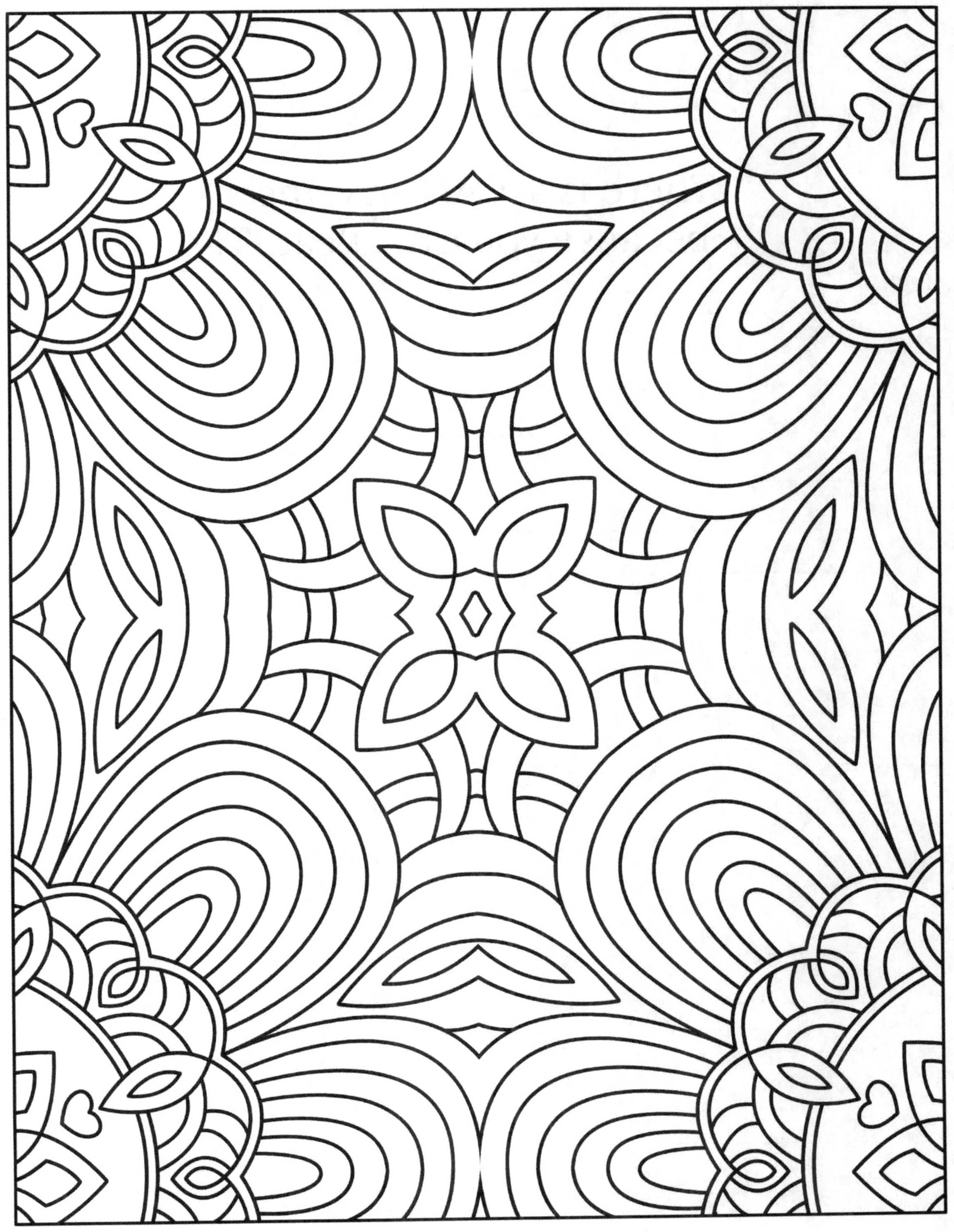

There is a 'CAN' in *Cancer*, because you CAN Beat IT!

Life may not be the party we hoped for, but while we are here we should *Dance!*

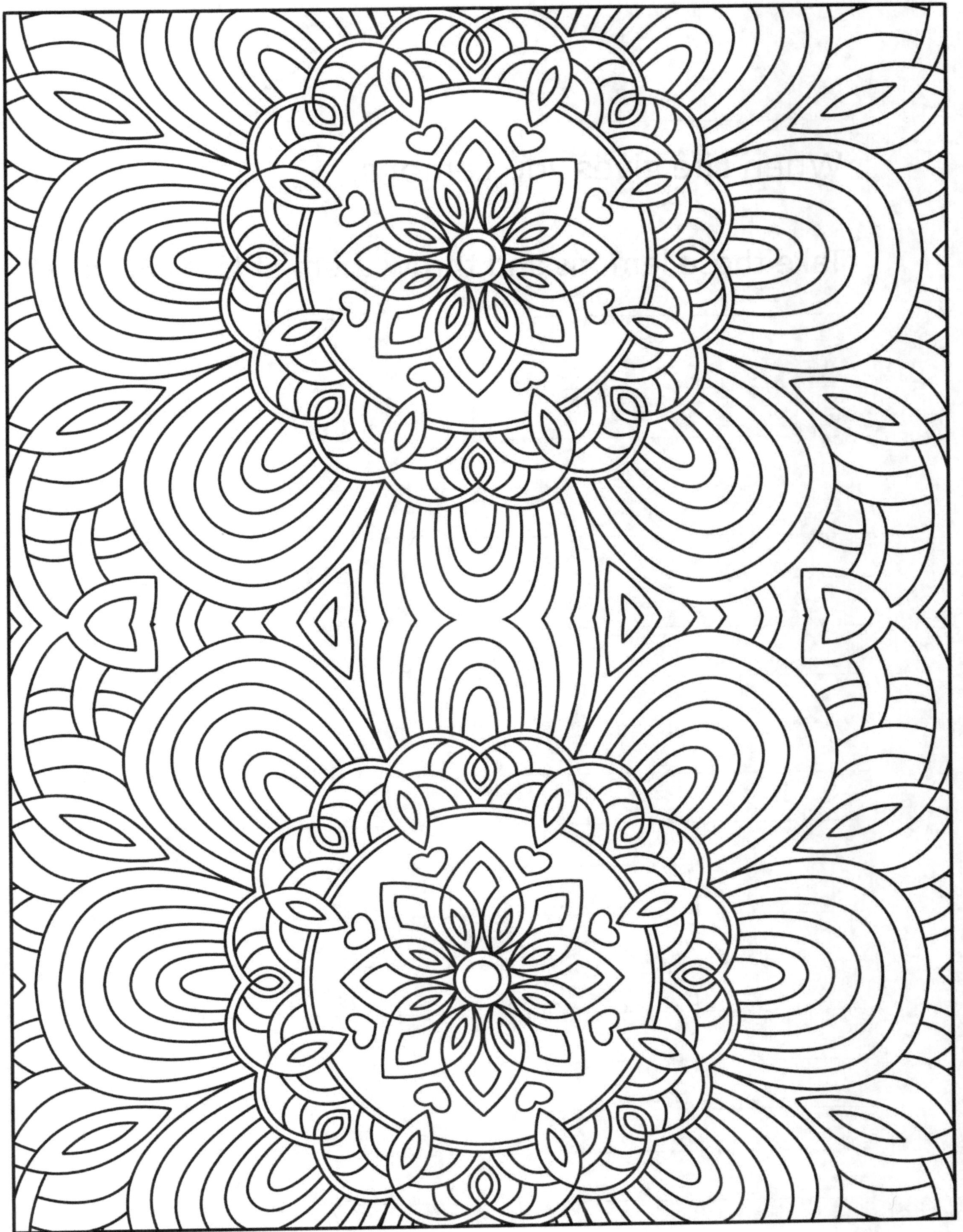

When Life gives you Lemons…

Take those lemons and throw them at Life's Balls!

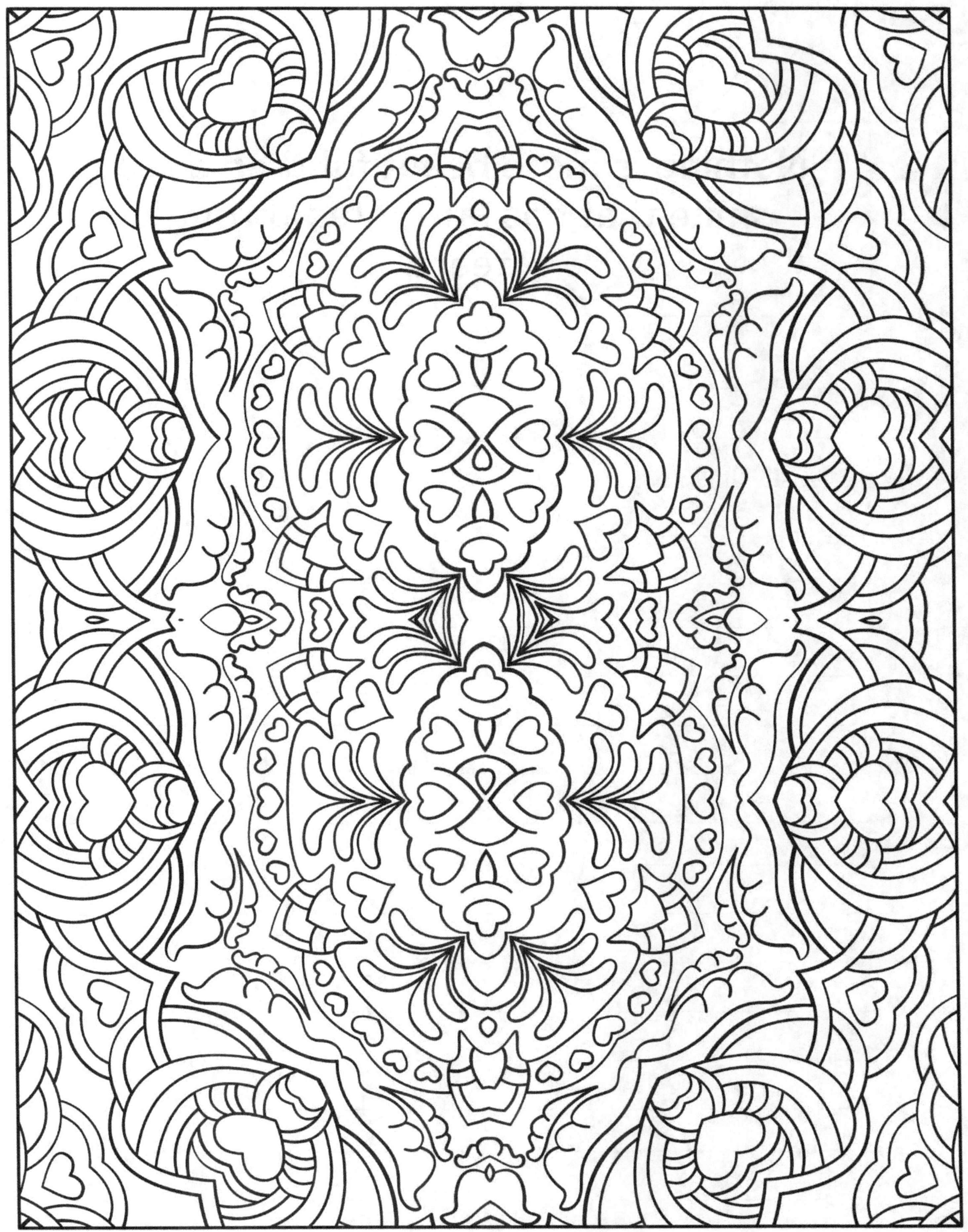

Nothing is more beautiful than a real smile that has struggled through tears.

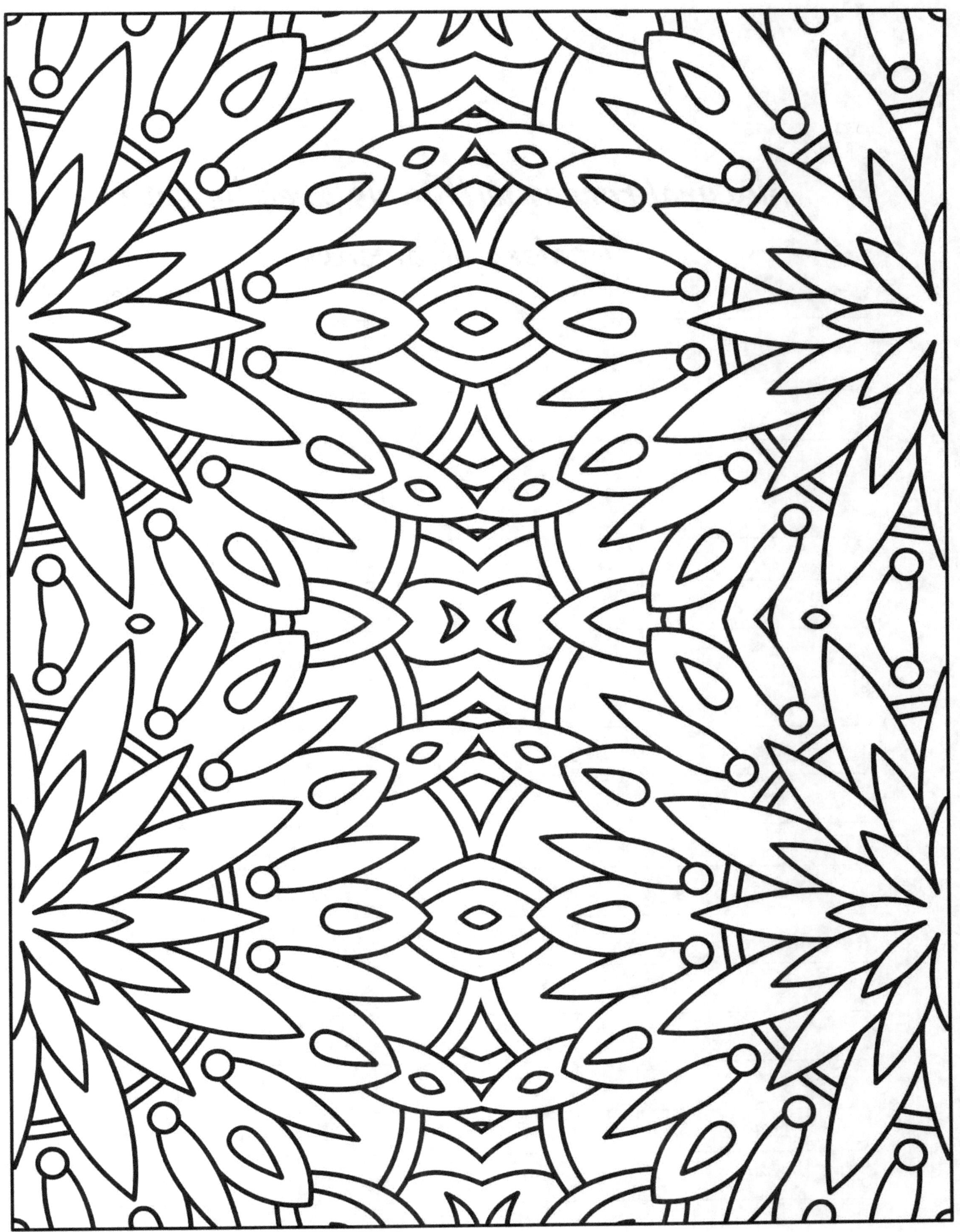

Natural forces within us are the true
healers of disease

Hippocrates

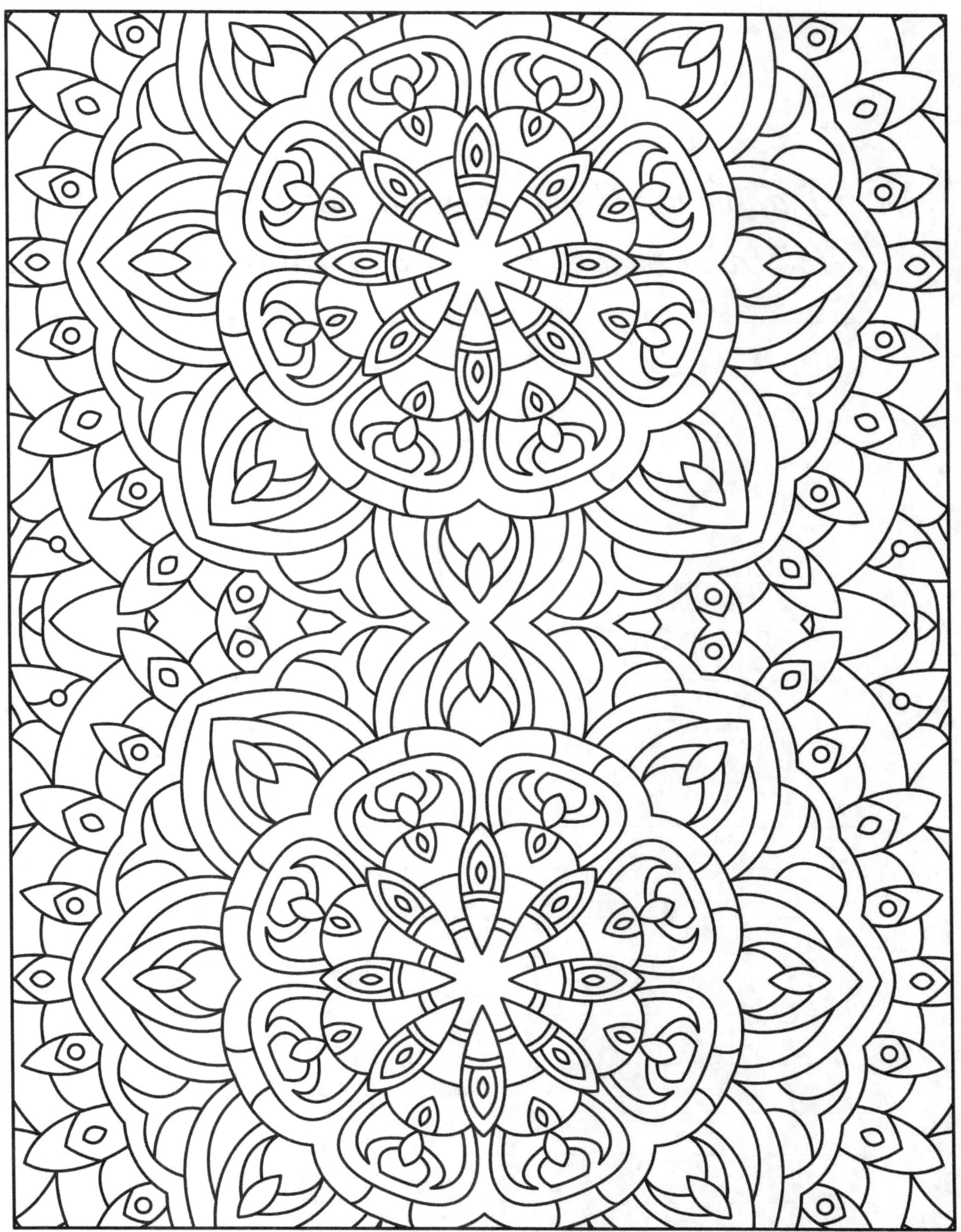

I don't want you to save me, I want you to stand beside me while I save myself!

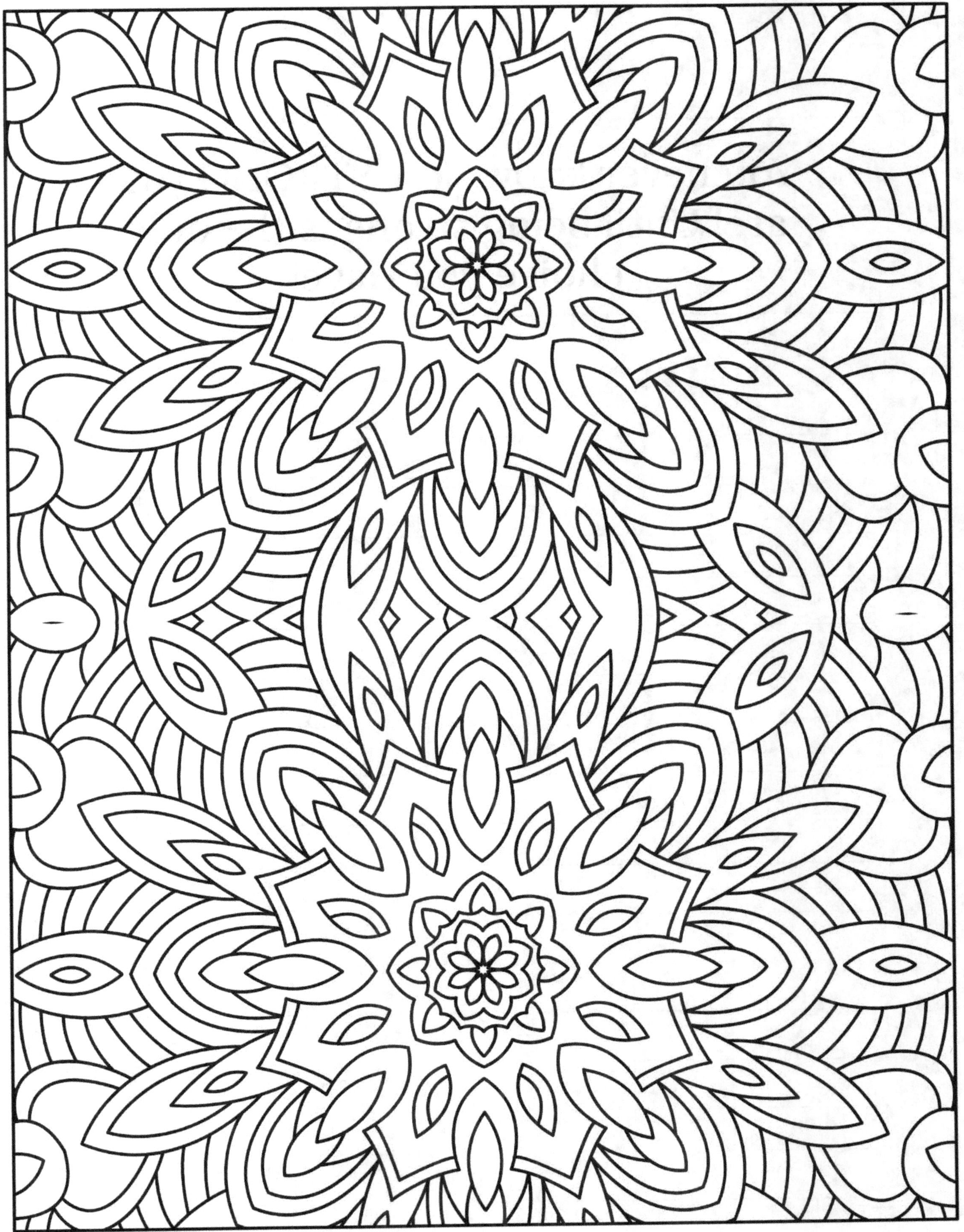

You never know how STRONG you are! Until being strong is the only choice you Have!

You have to fight through some bad days to get to the best days!

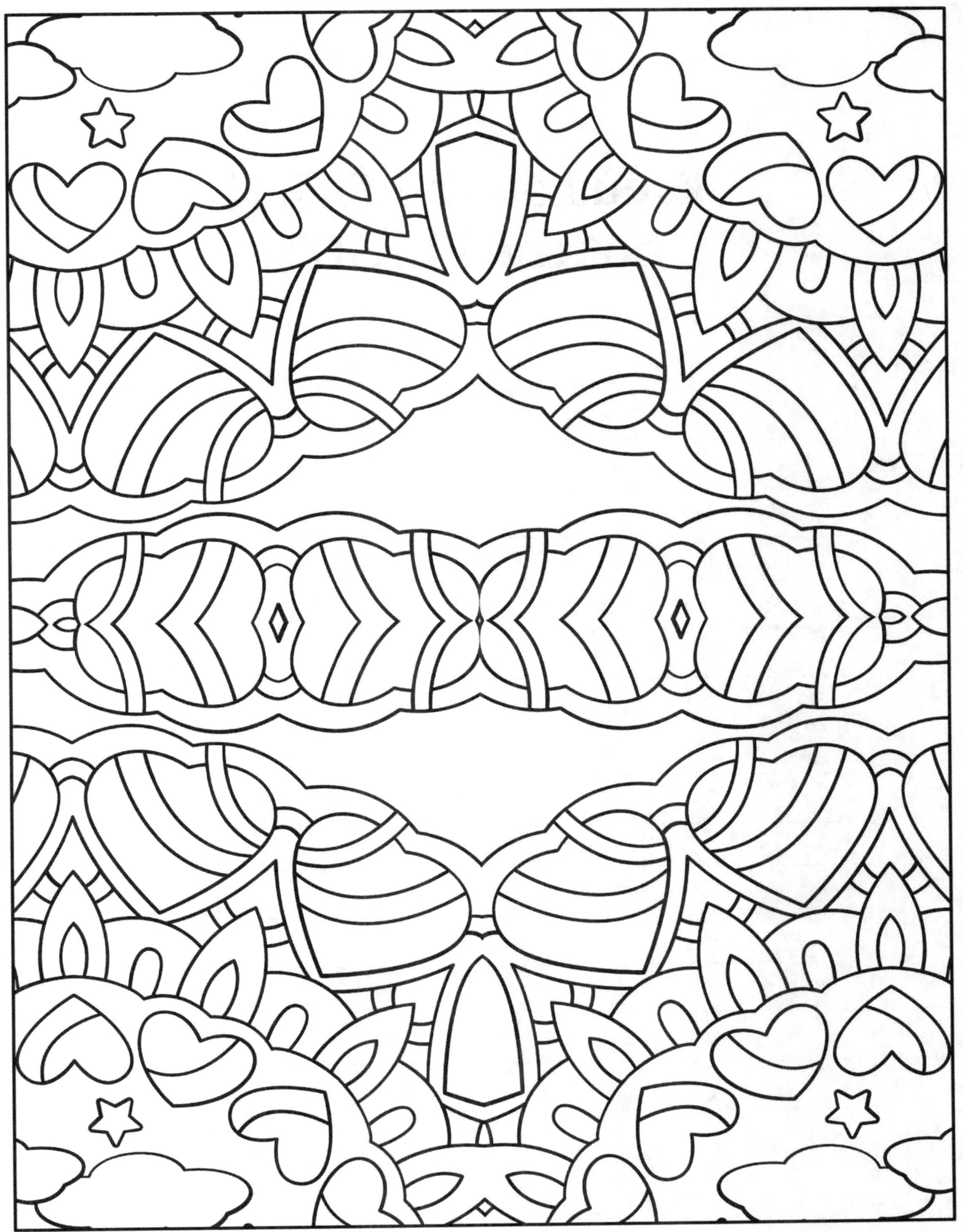

Focus on the FIGHT
not the FRIGHT!

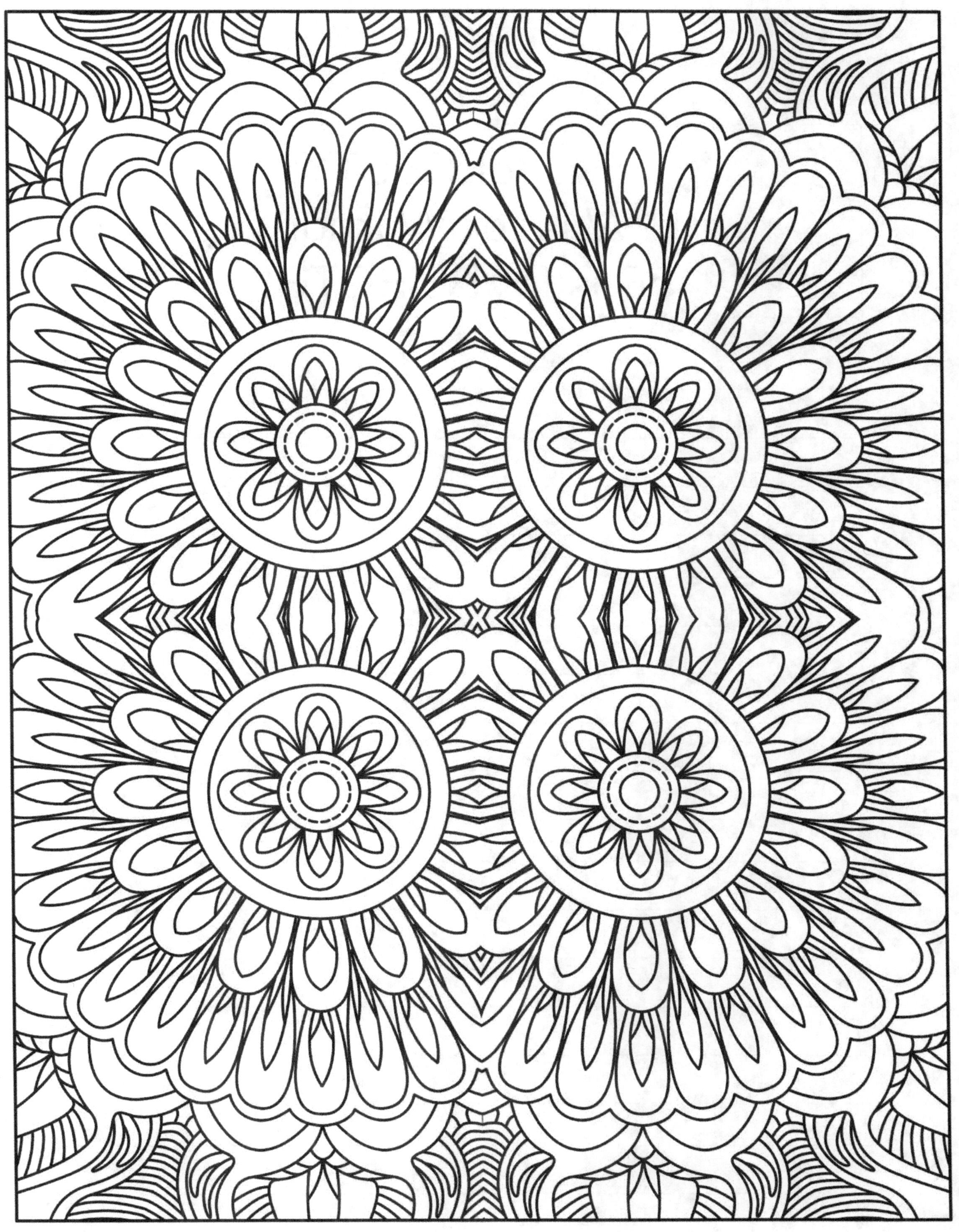

F is for FEISTY!
W is for Warrior!
B is for BE BOTH!

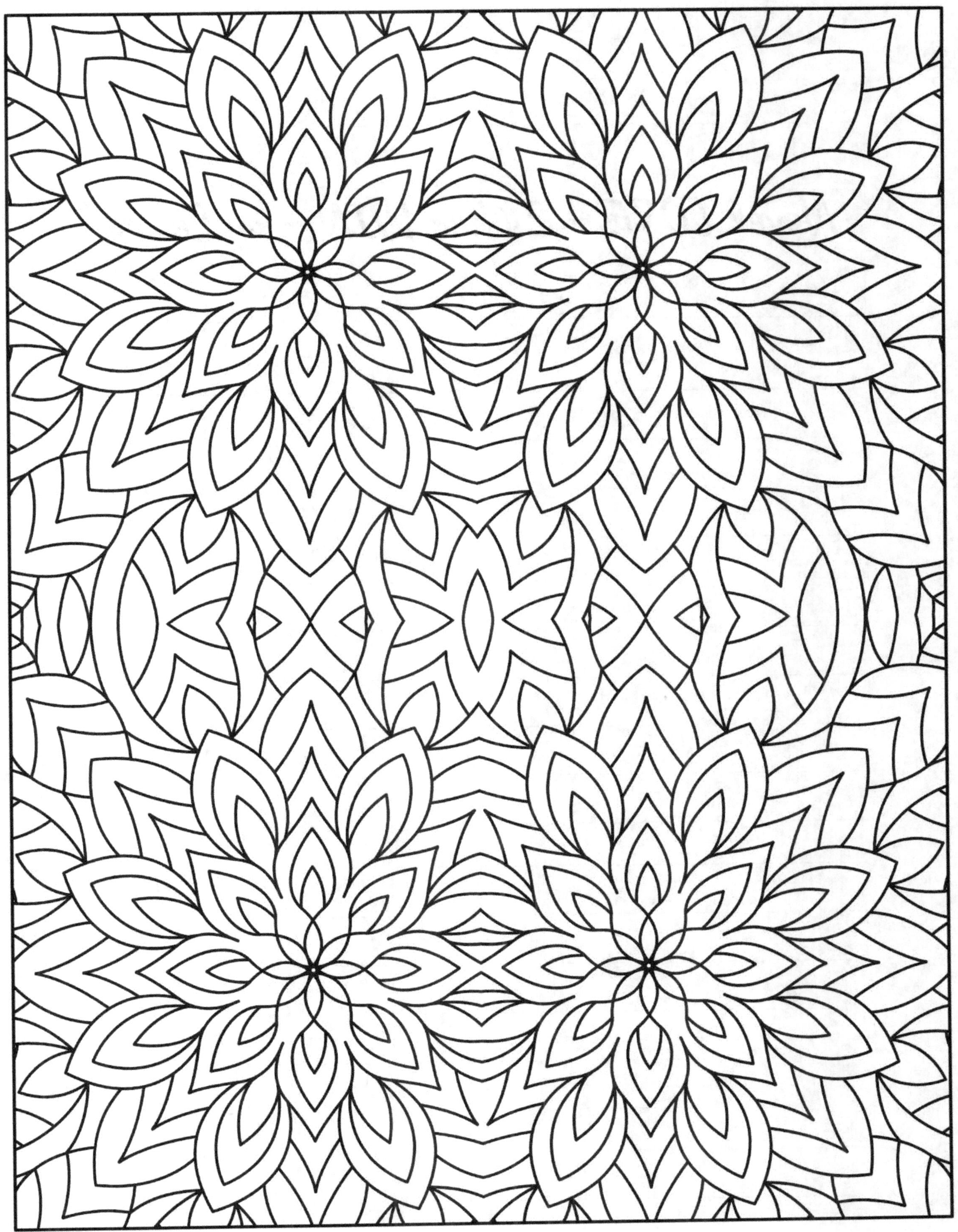

Never LOSE ~ Either WIN ~ or Learn!

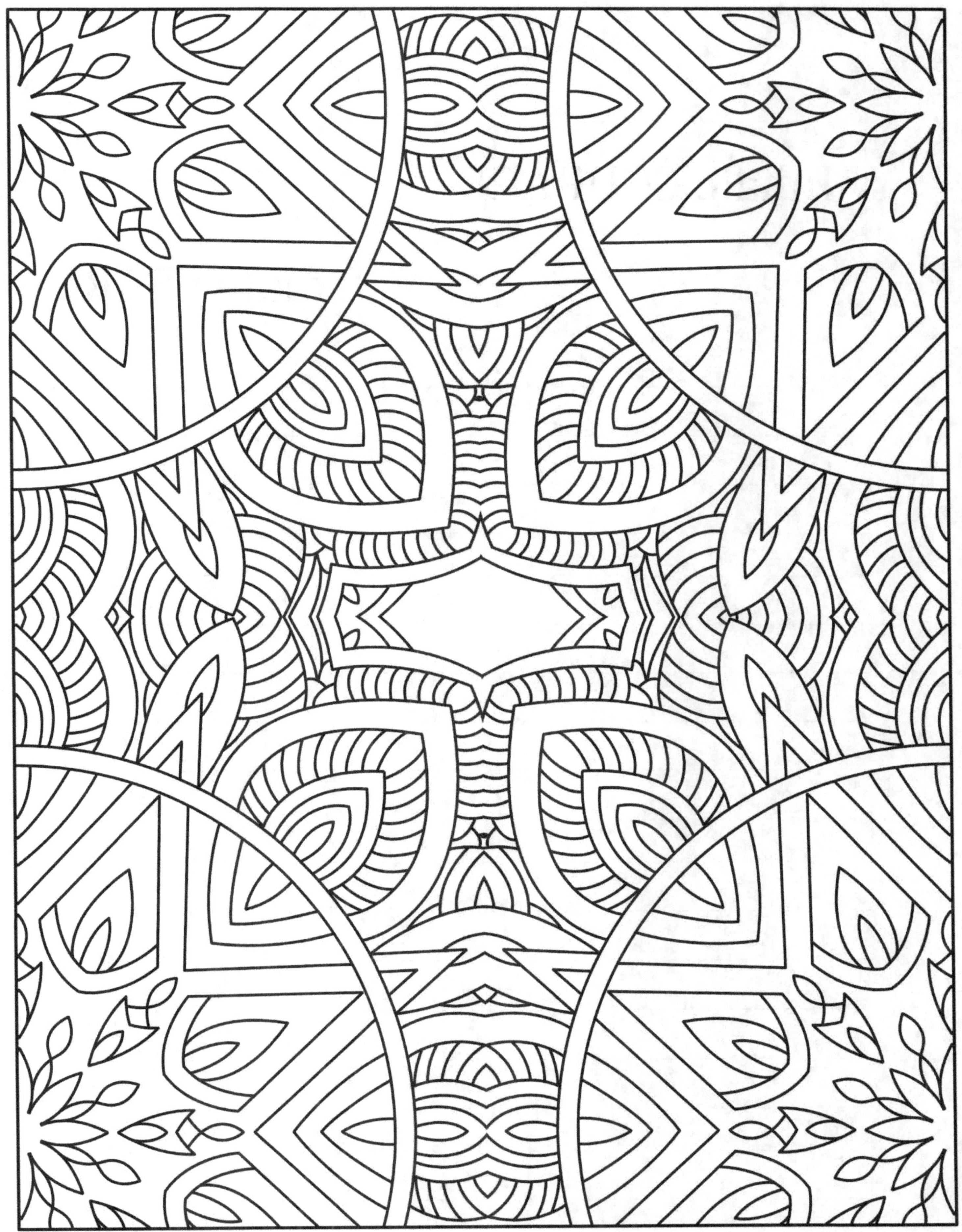

Inhale COURAGE….

...Exhale FEAR!

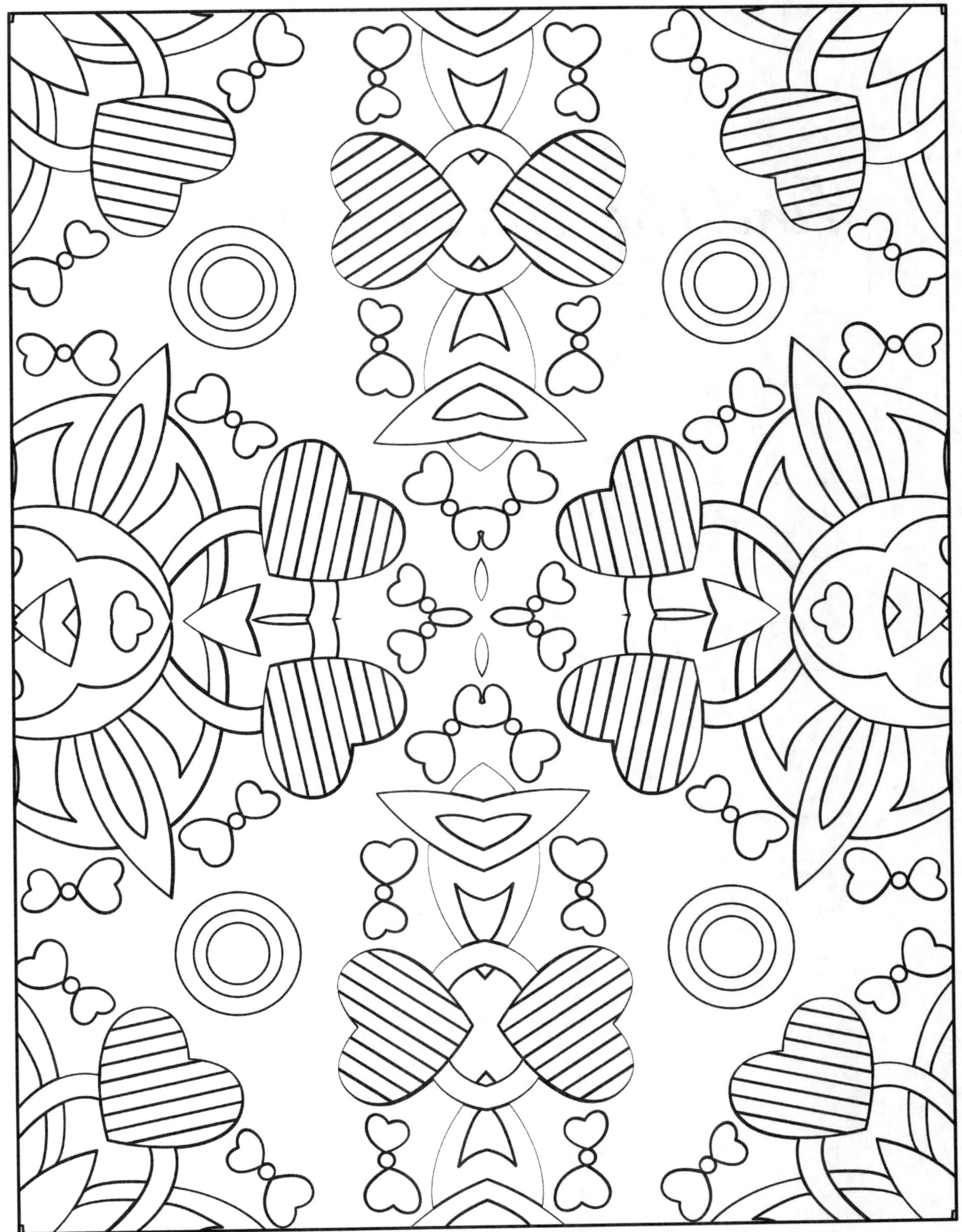

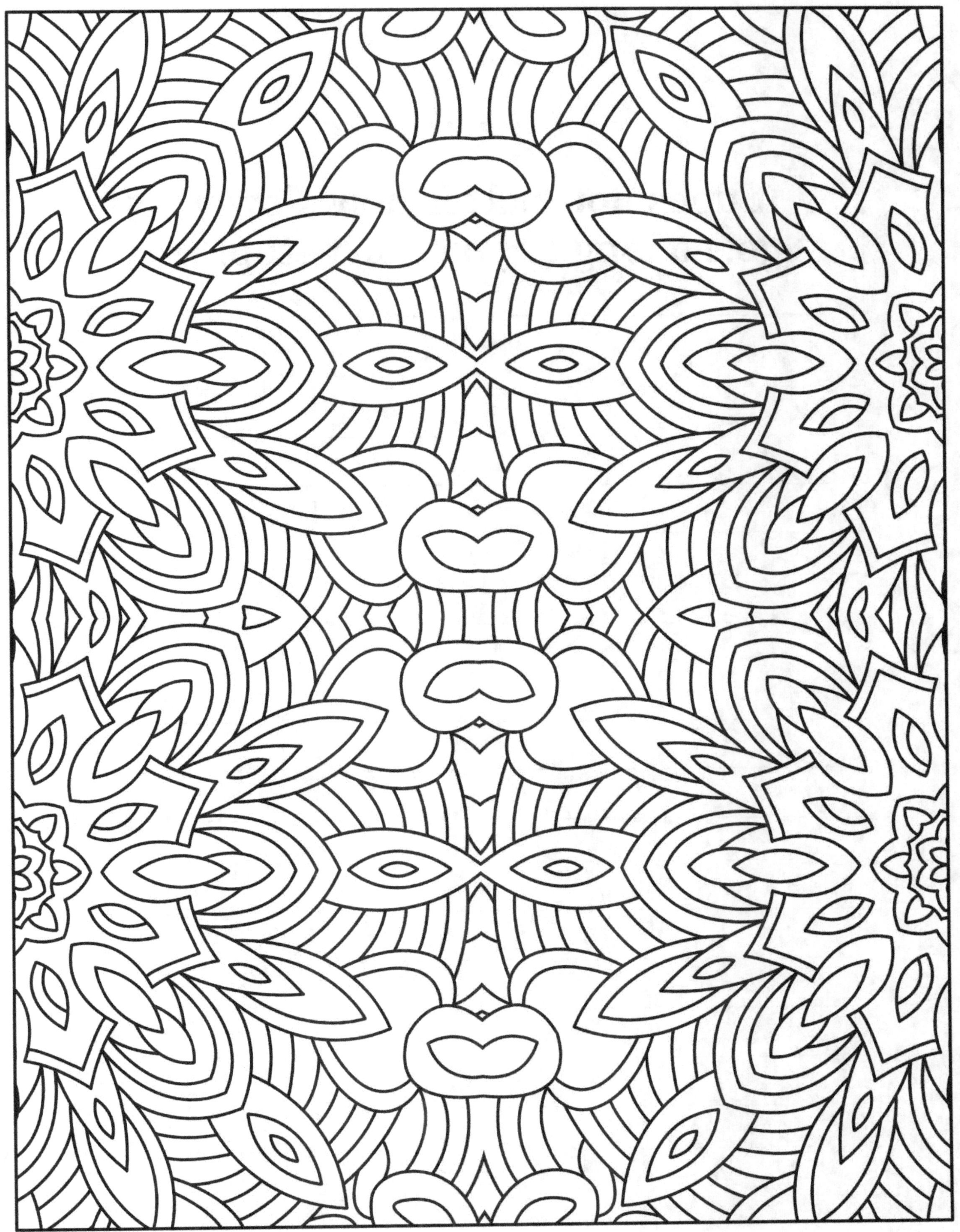

It does not matter how slowly you go, so long as you don't stop!

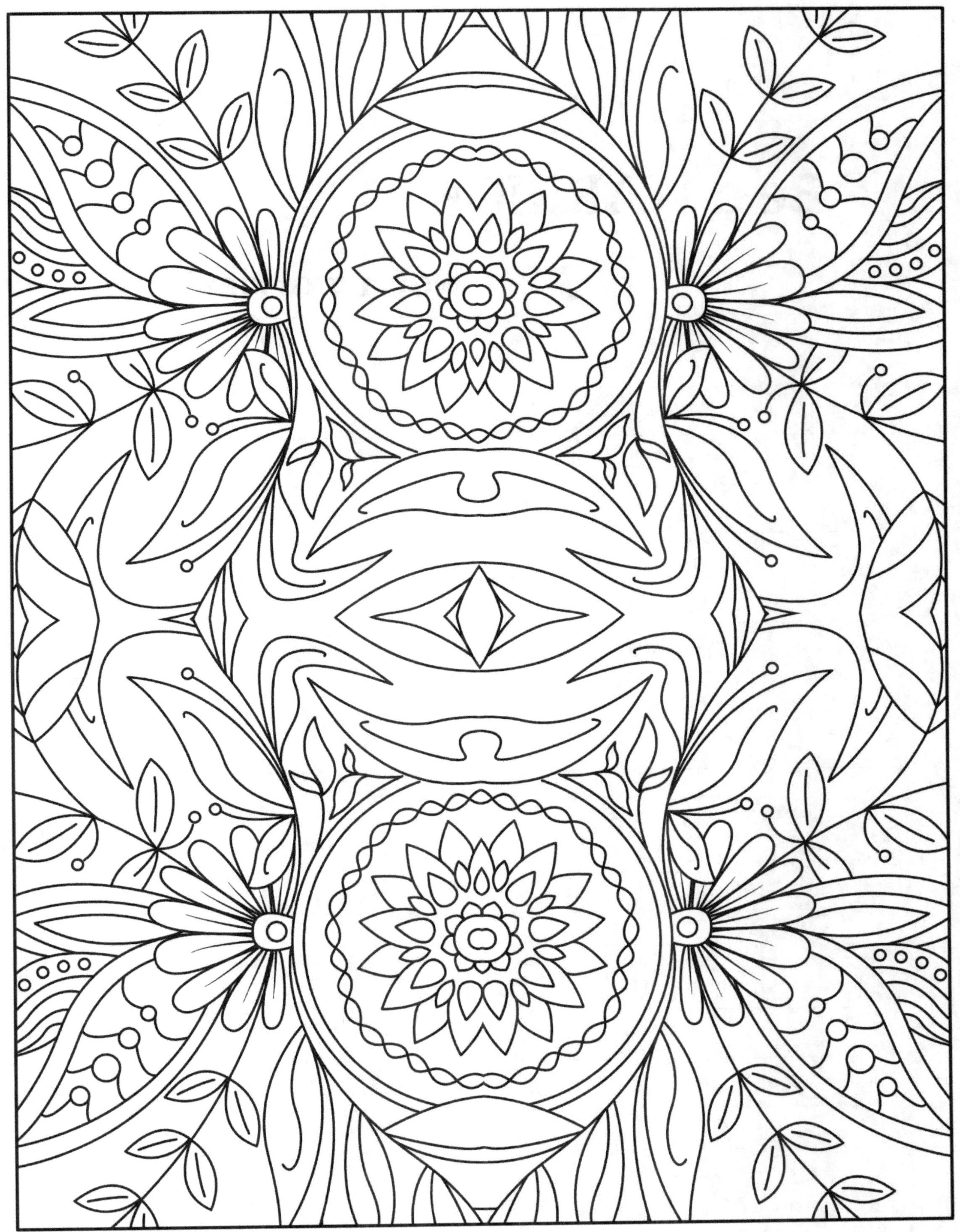

Be a WARRIOR

Not a worrier!

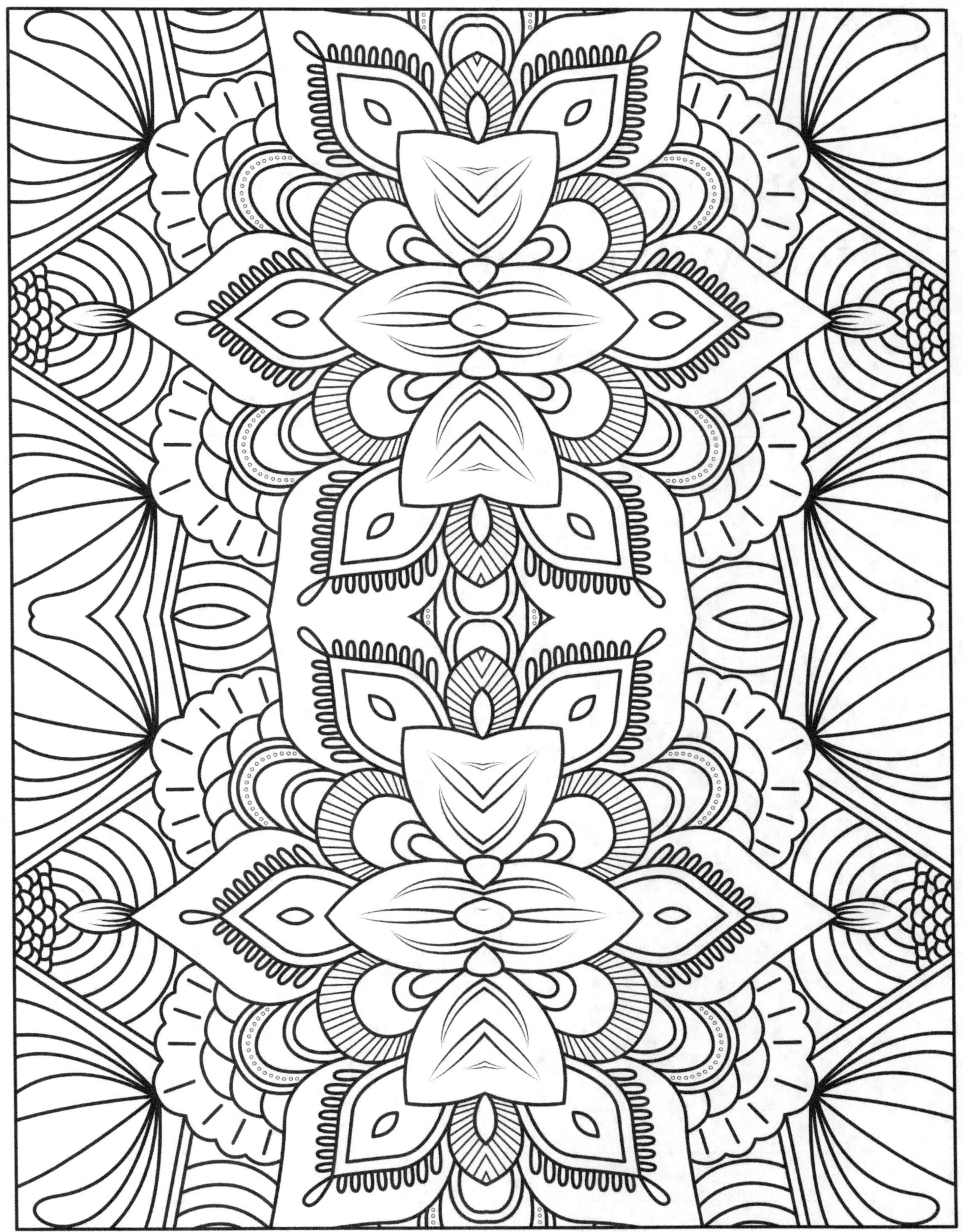

You may see me struggle, but you will never see me quit!

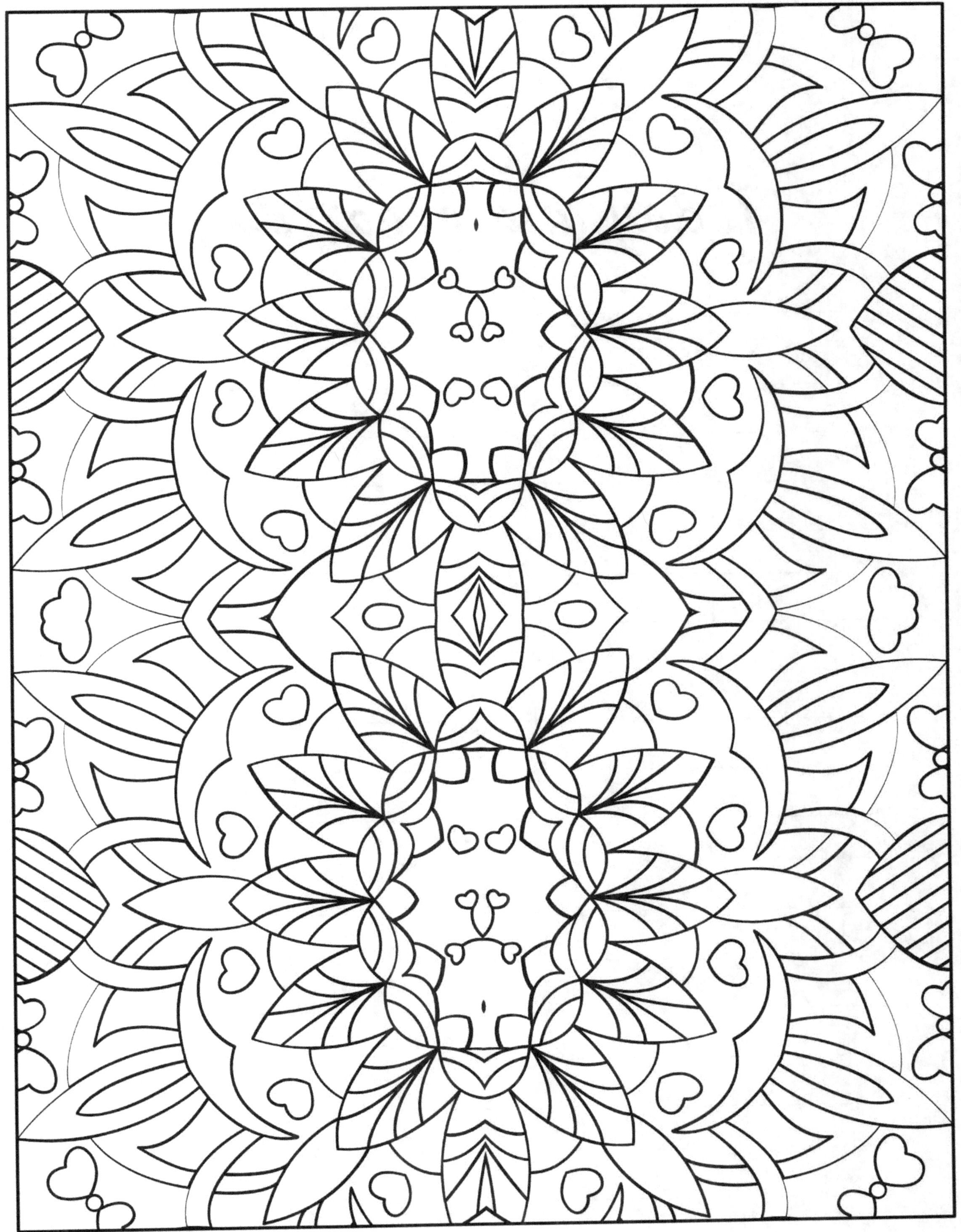

Today is a great day!

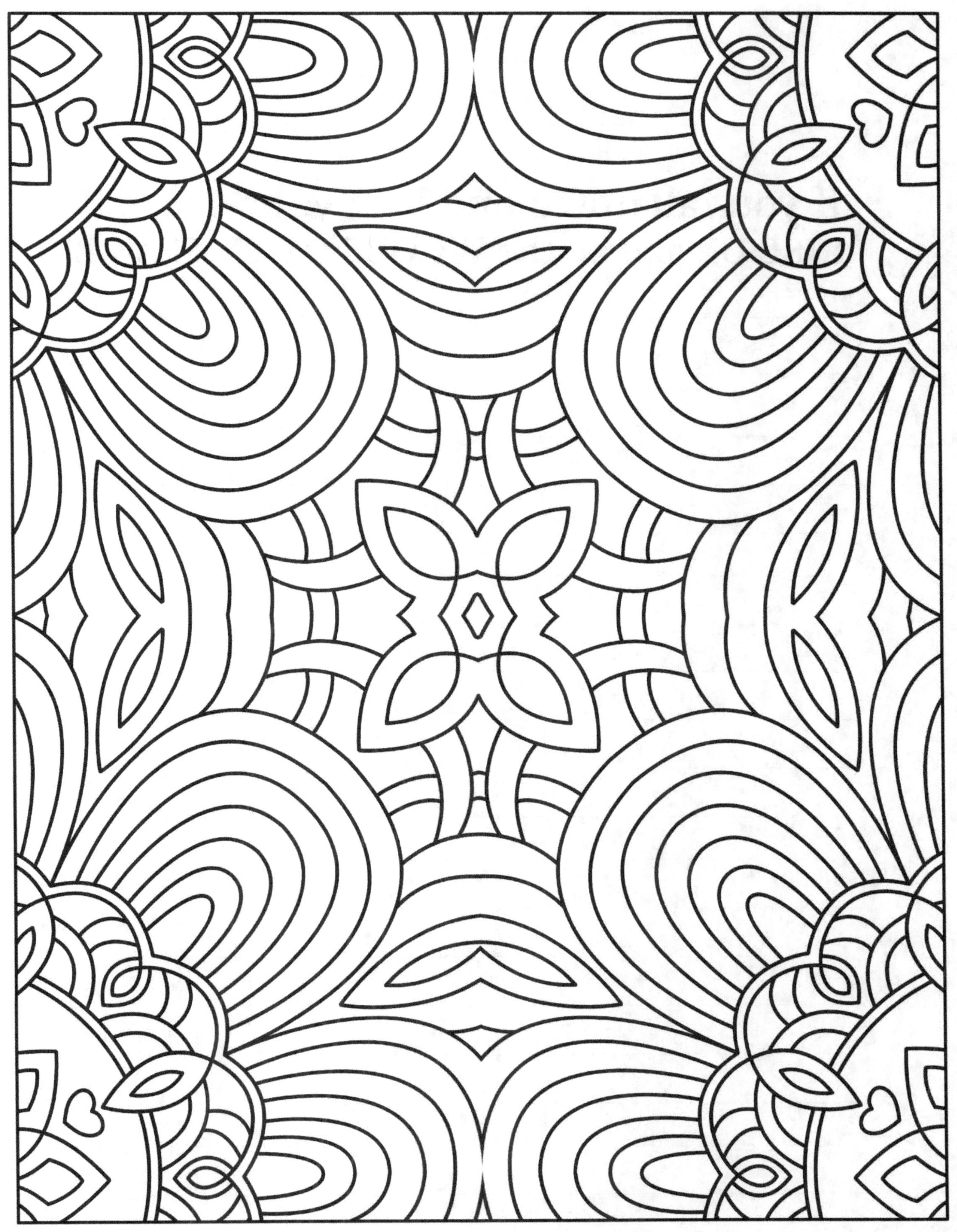

If you fall down and lose your spark...
RISE UP and be the WHOLE DAMN FLAME!

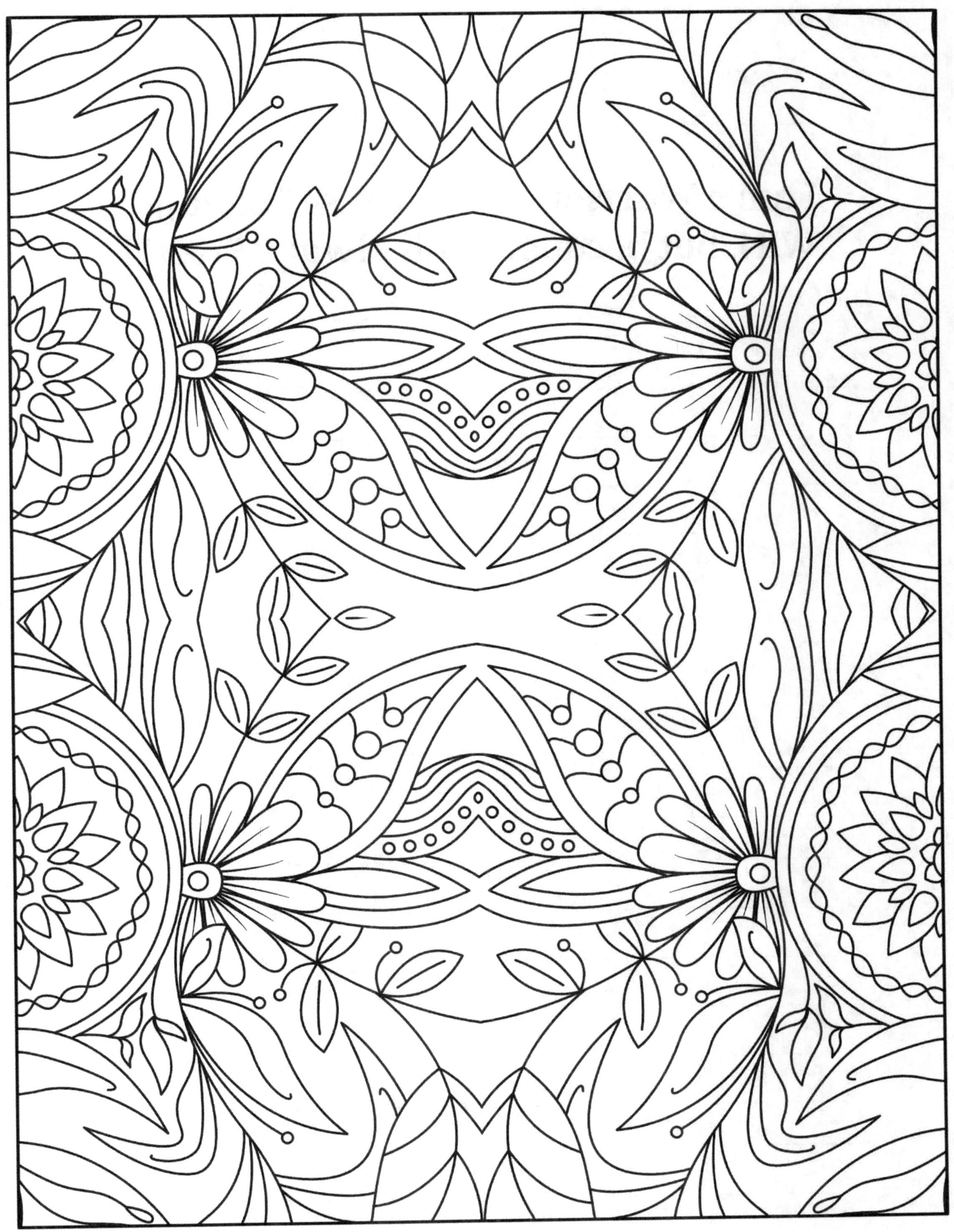

I am a Warrior! Not because I always WIN, but because I will always FIGHT!

You're a Warrior, and Warriors Don't Quit. Cancer Is Just One Chapter in Your Life, Not the Whole Story.

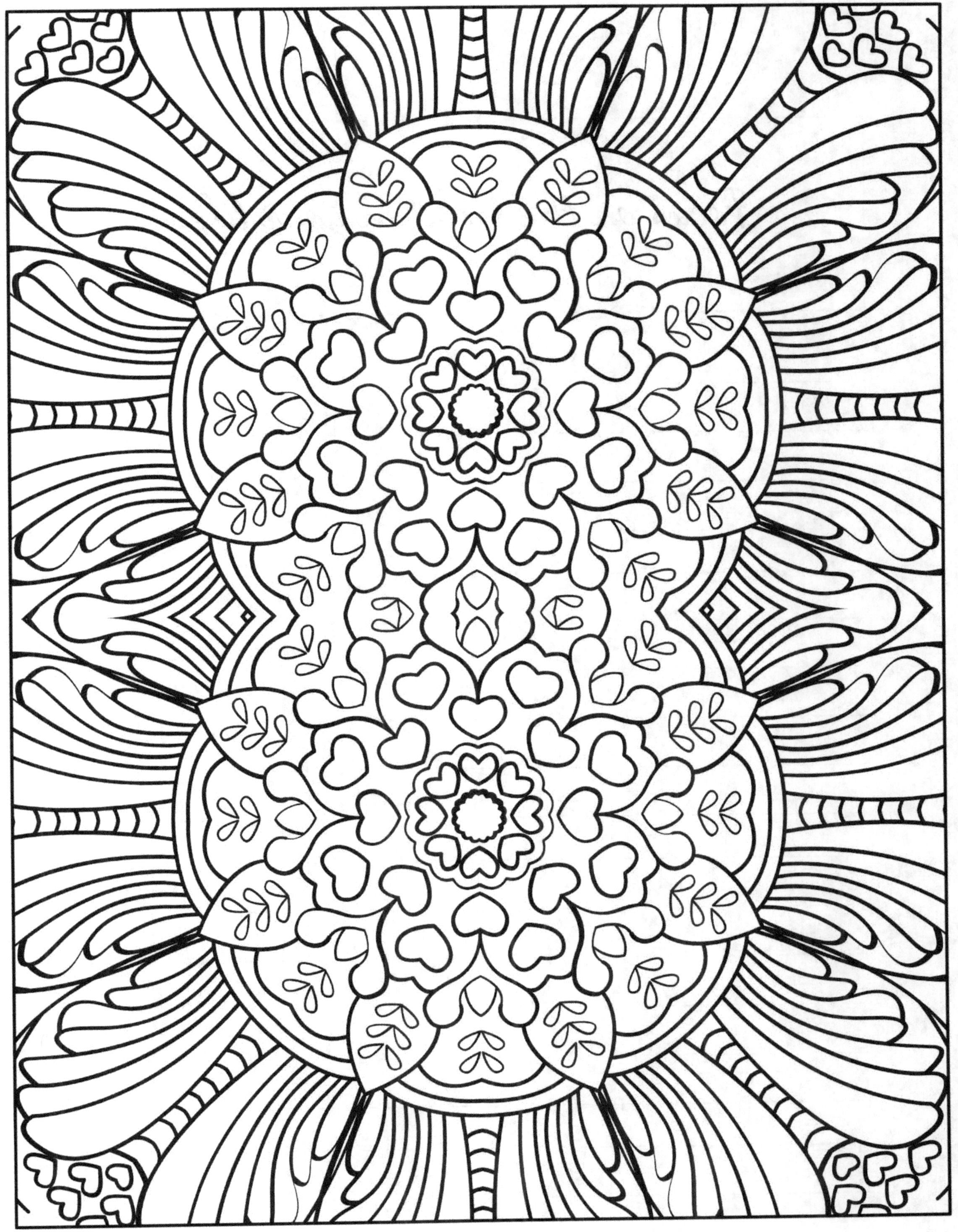

Focus on the Good in your life.

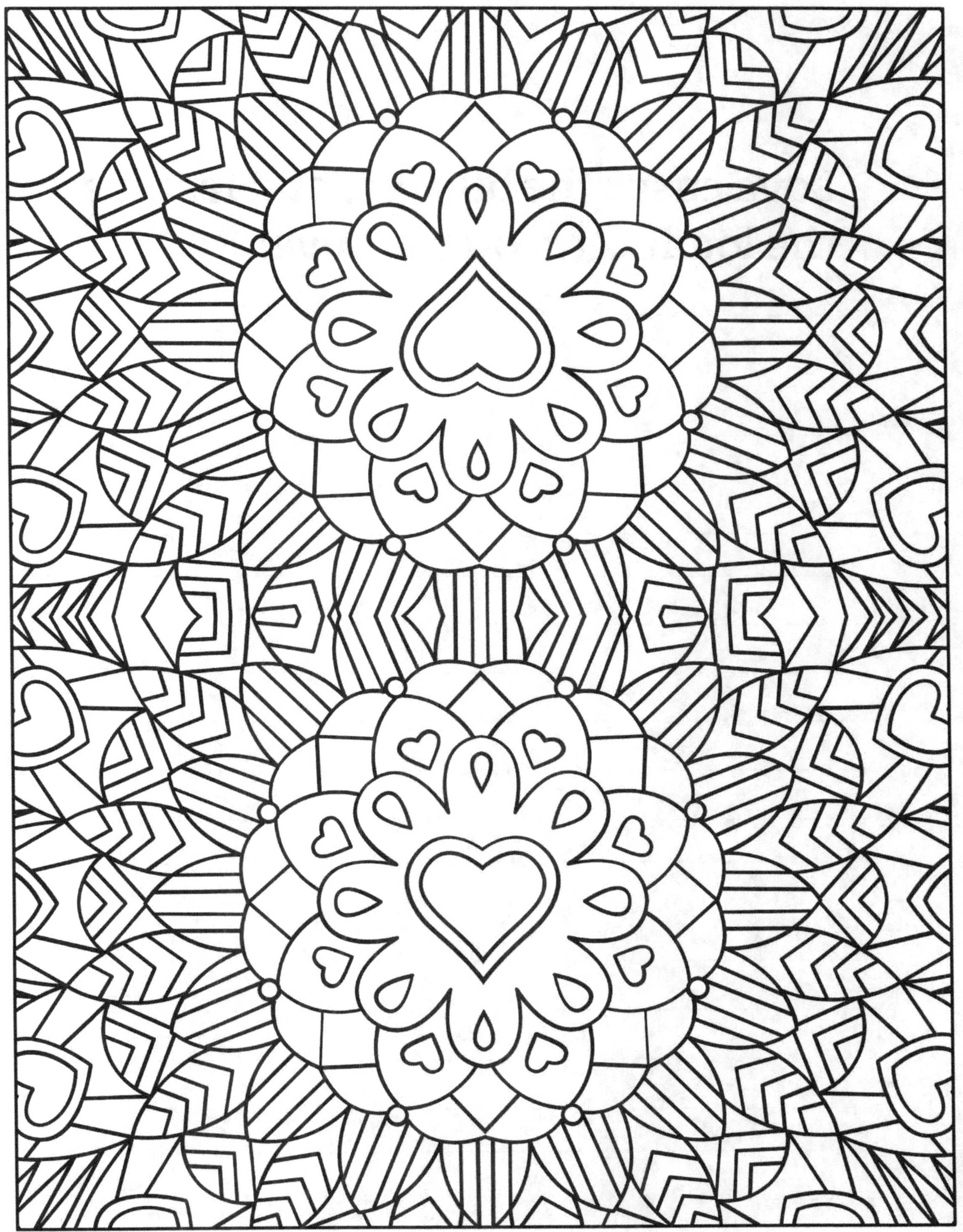

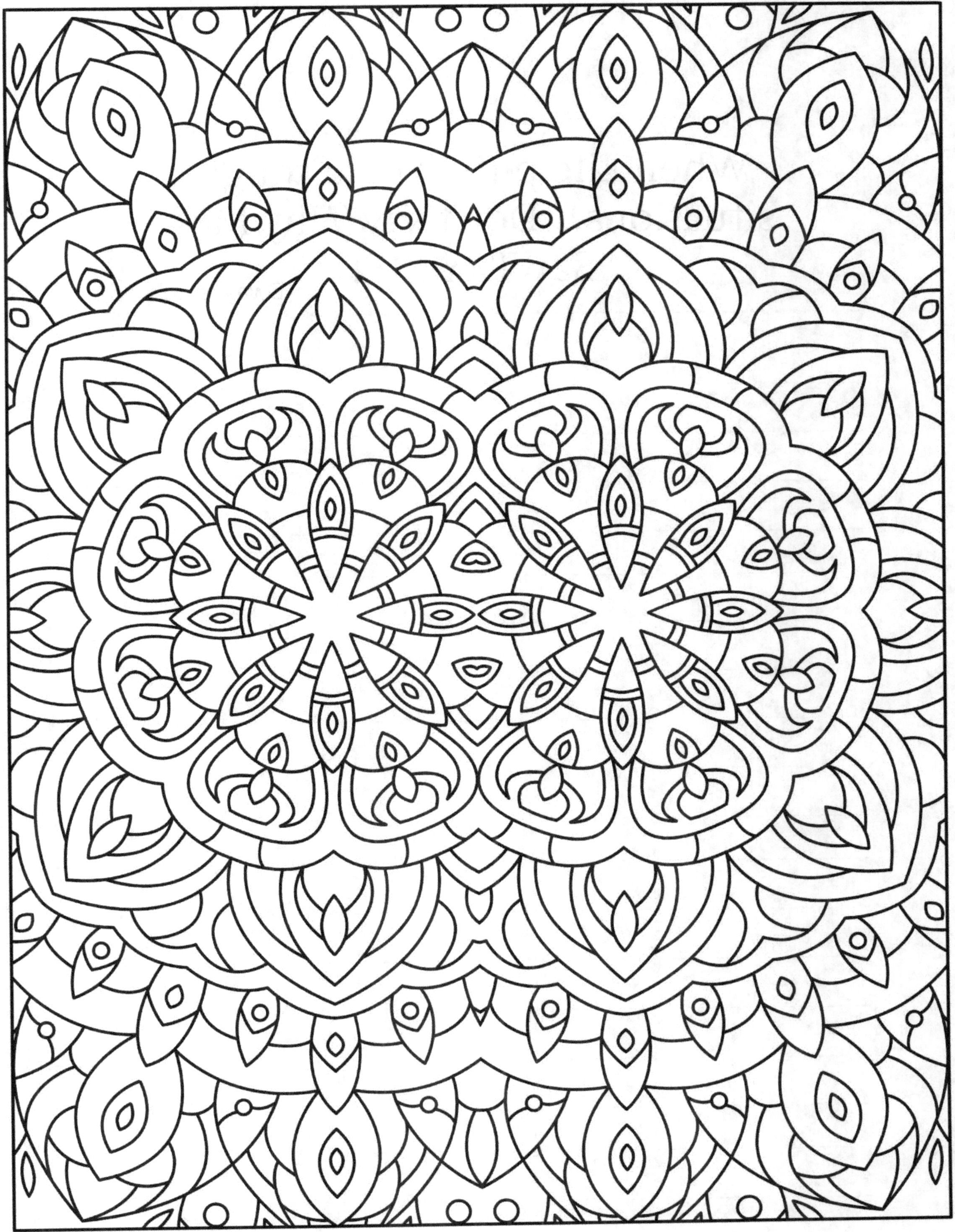

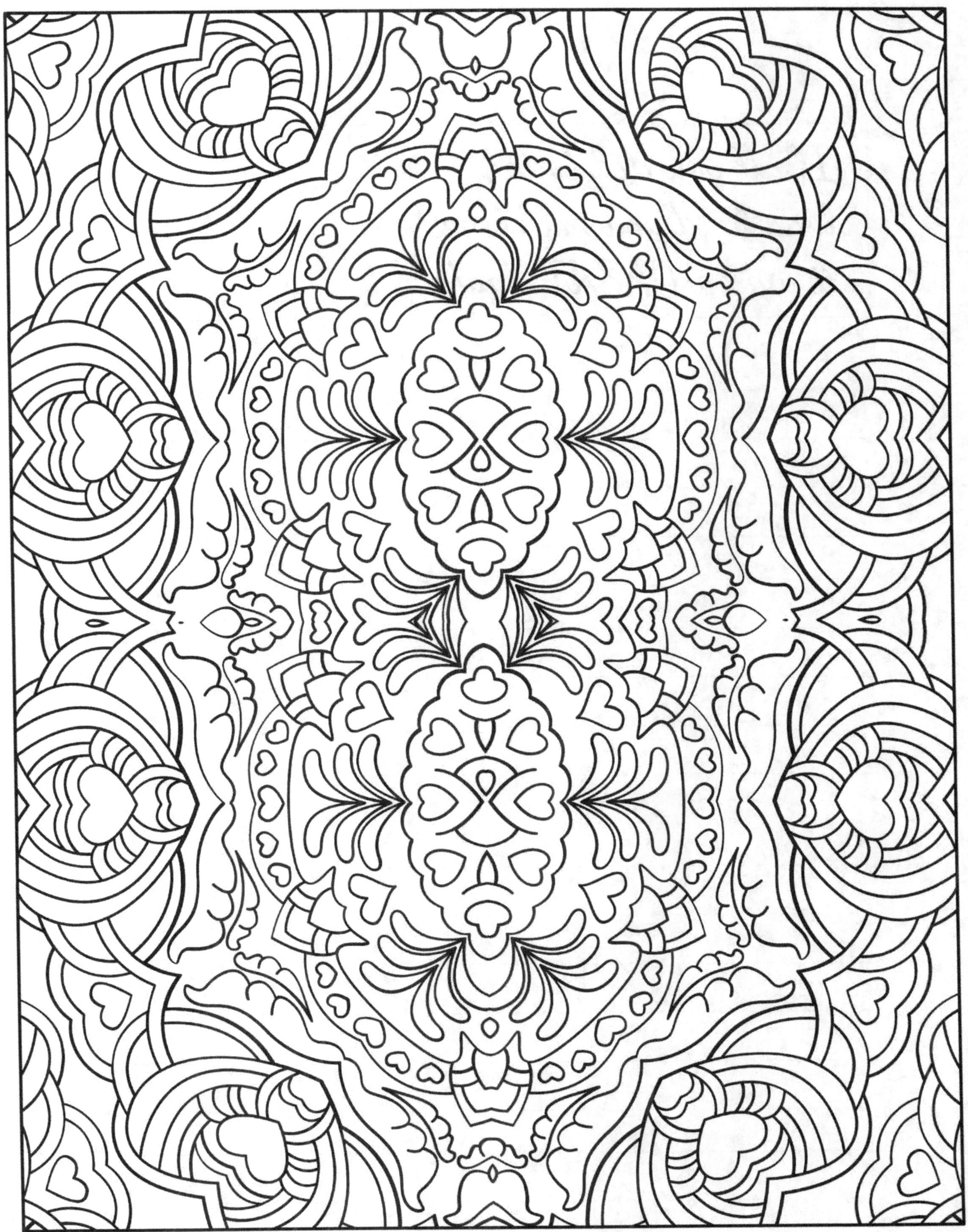

If all you did today...
was hold yourself together...
it was a GREAT day!

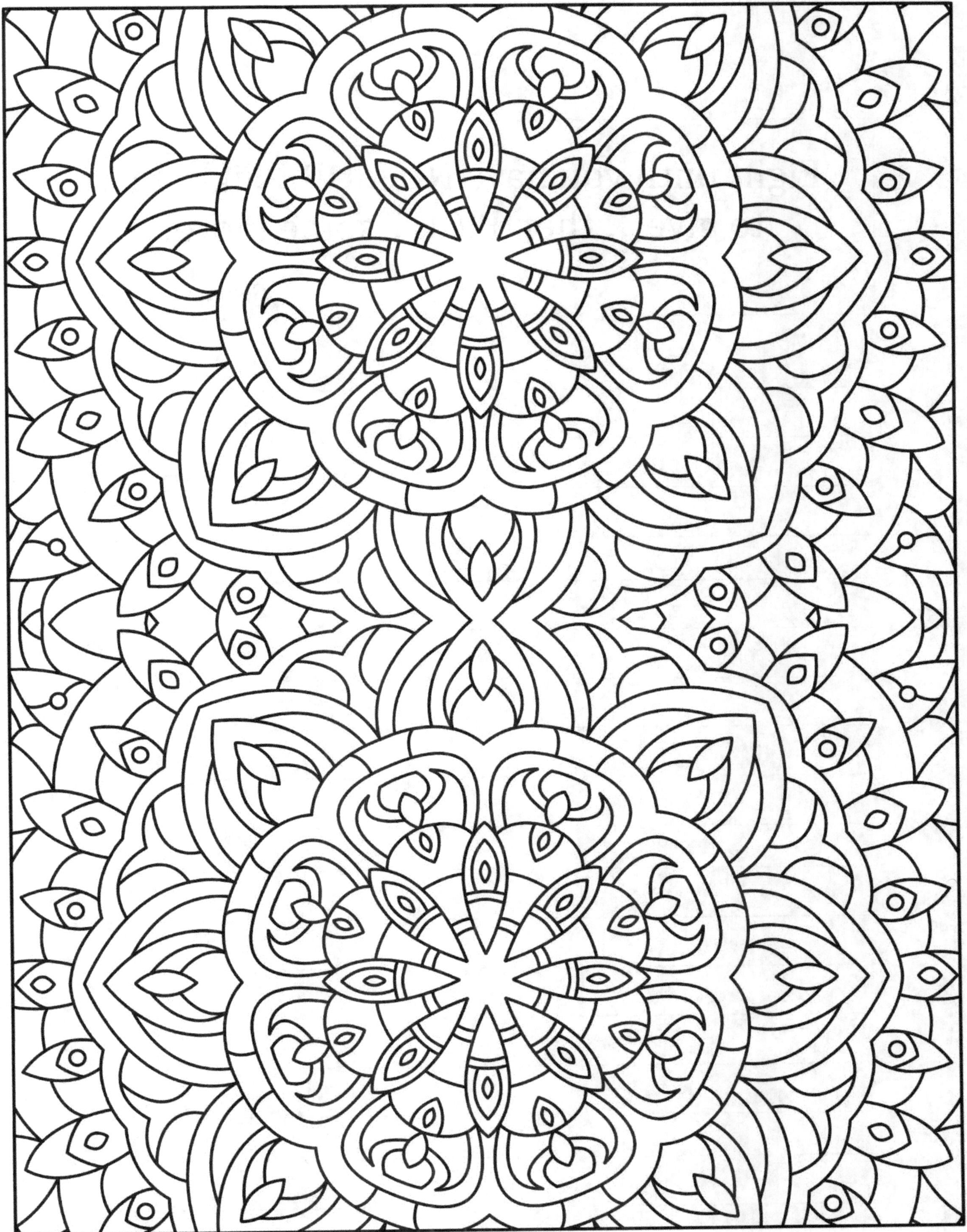

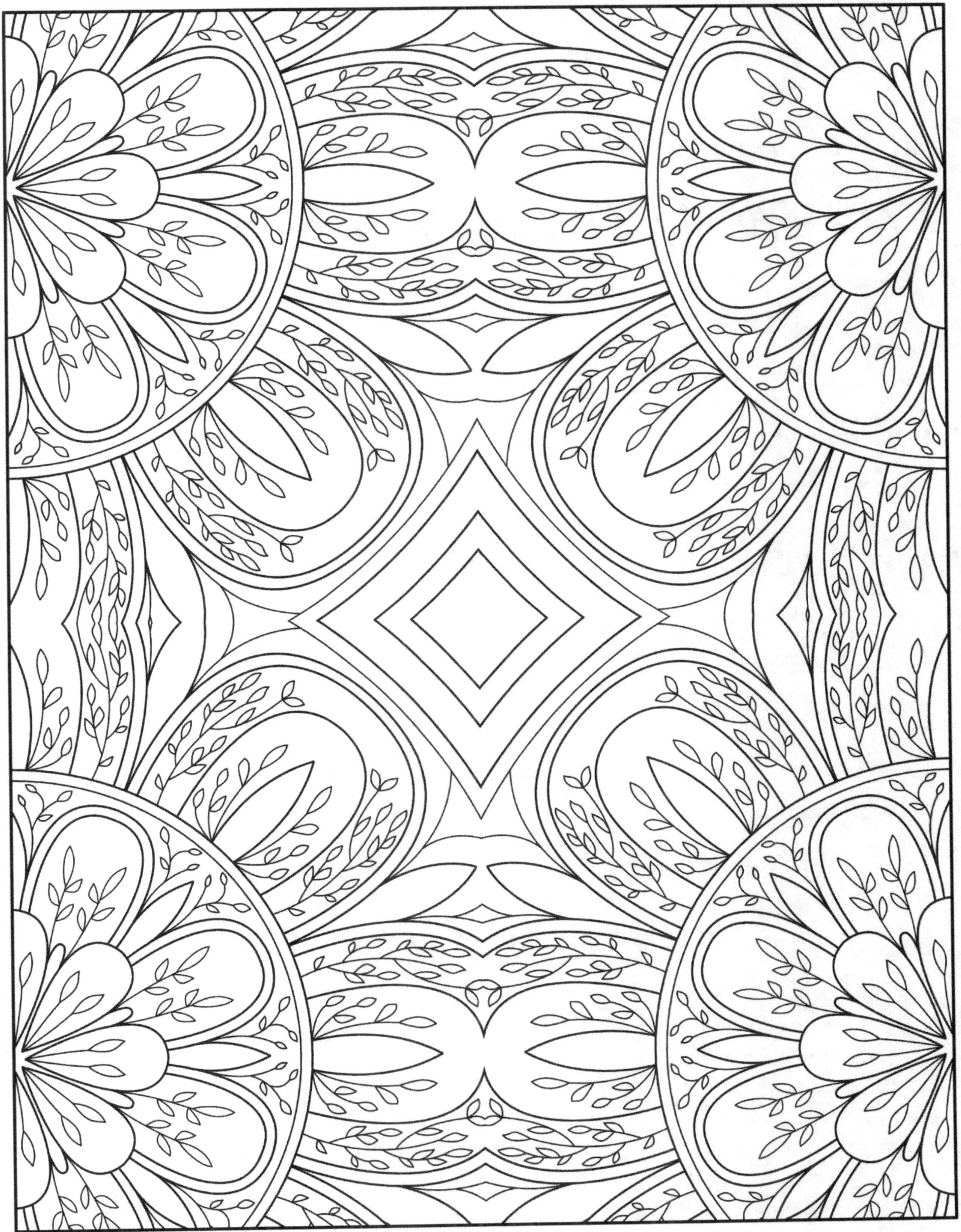

Allow yourself to be humble

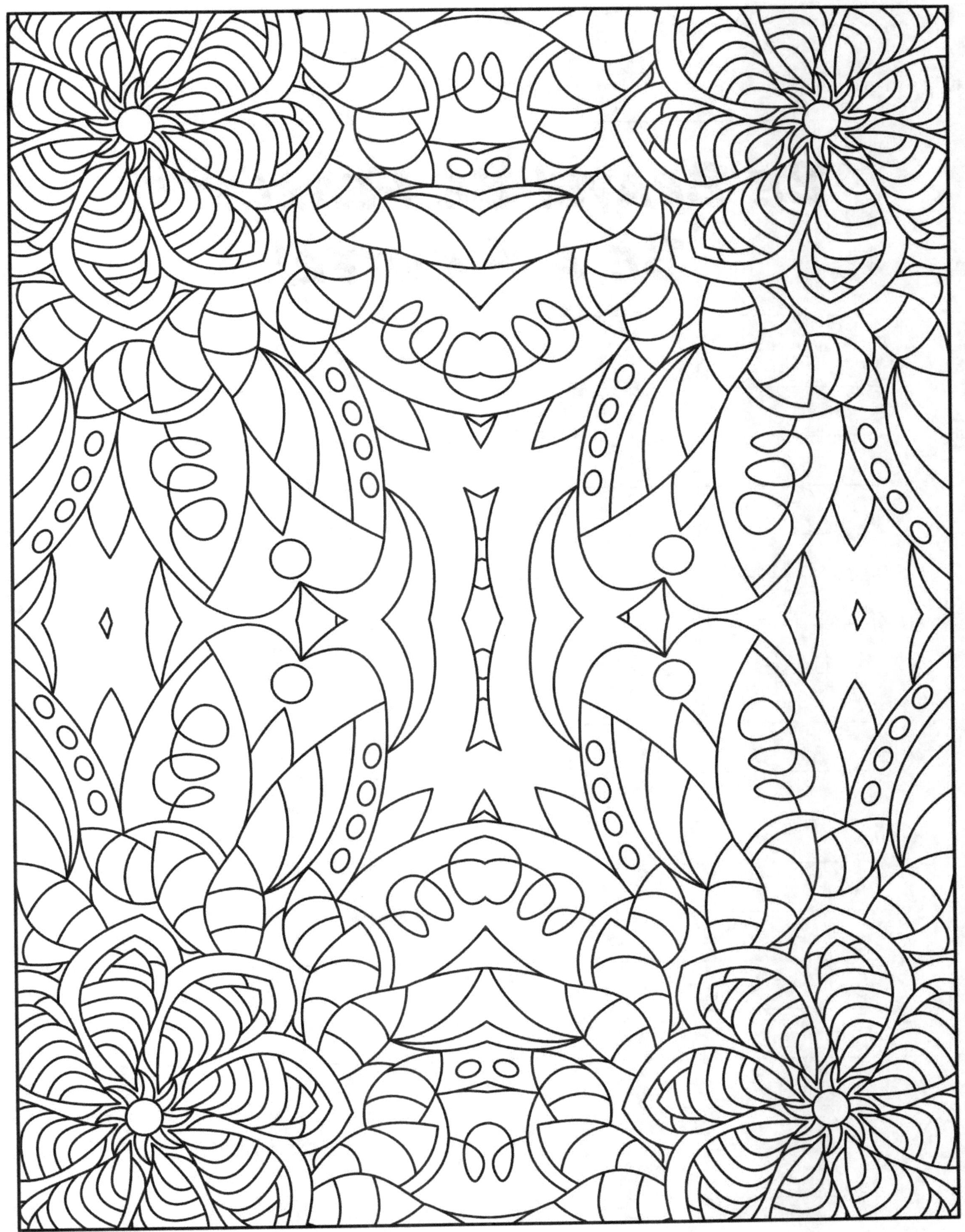

Be Brave! Be Fearless! Be a Fighter!